& Answers
About Head and
Brain Injuries

Rahul Jandial, MD, PhD

Assistant Professor
Division of Neurological Surgery
City of Hope Cancer Center
Los Angeles, CA

Charles B. Newman, MD

Resident Neurosurgeon
University of California, San Diego
Division of Neurological Surgery

Samuel A. Hughes, MD, PhD

Resident Neurosurgeon
Oregon Health & Science University
Department of Neurological Surgery

JONES AND BARTLETT PUBLISHERS

Sudbury, Massachusetts

BOSTON   TORONTO   LONDON   SINGAPORE

World Headquarters
Jones and Bartlett Publishers
40 Tall Pine Drive
Sudbury, MA 01776
978-443-5000
info@jbpub.com
www.jbpub.com

Jones and Bartlett Publishers
Canada
6339 Ormindale Way
Mississauga, Ontario L5V 1J2
Canada

Jones and Bartlett Publishers
International
Barb House, Barb Mews
London W6 7PA
United Kingdom

Jones and Bartlett's books and products are available through most bookstores and online booksellers. To contact Jones and Bartlett Publishers directly, call 800-832-0034, fax 978-443-8000, or visit our website, www.jbpub.com.

Substantial discounts on bulk quantities of Jones and Bartlett's publications are available to corporations, professional associations, and other qualified organizations. For details and specific discount information, contact the special sales department at Jones and Bartlett via the above contact information or send an email to specialsales@jbpub.com.

The authors, editor, and publisher have made every effort to provide accurate information. However, they are not responsible for errors, omissions, or for any outcomes related to the use of the contents of this book and take no responsibility for the use of the products and procedures described. Treatments and side effects described in this book may not be applicable to all people; likewise, some people may require a dose or experience a side effect that is not described herein. Drugs and medical devices are discussed that may have limited availability controlled by the Food and Drug Administration (FDA) for use only in a research study or clinical trial. Research, clinical practice, and government regulations often change the accepted standard in this field. When consideration is being given to use of any drug in the clinical setting, the health care provider or reader is responsible for determining FDA status of the drug, reading the package insert, and reviewing prescribing information for the most up-to-date recommendations on dose, precautions, and contraindications, and determining the appropriate usage for the product. This is especially important in the case of drugs that are new or seldom used.

Production Credits
Executive Publisher: Christopher Davis
Production Director: Amy Rose
Associate Editor: Kathy Richardson
Sr. Editorial Assistant: Jessica Acox
Associate Production Editor: Leah Corrigan
V.P., Manufacturing and Inventory Control:
    Therese Connell

Associate Marketing Manager: Ilana Goddess
Composition: Lynn L'Heureux
Cover Design: Carolyn Downer
Printing and Binding: Malloy, Inc.
Cover Printing: Malloy, Inc.
Cover Images: © Jerry Sharp/ShutterStock, Inc.
    © Amy Myers/ShutterStock, Inc.
    © E. Dygas/Photodisc/Getty Images

Library of Congress Cataloging-in-Publication Data
Jandial, Rahul.
  100 questions & answers about head and brain injuries / Rahul Jandial.
    p. ; cm.
  Includes bibliographical references.
  ISBN 978-0-7637-5572-0 (alk. paper)
  1. Brain damage--Miscellanea. 2. Brain damage--Popular works. 3. Head--Wounds and injuries--Miscellanea. 4. Head--Wounds and injuries--Popular works. I. Title. II. Title: One hundred Questions & Answers about head and brain injuries.
  [DNLM: 1. Craniocerebral Trauma--diagnosis--Examination Questions. 2. Craniocerebral Trauma--therapy--Examination Questions. WL 18.2 J33z 2009]
  RC387.5.J36 2009
  617.4'81044--dc22

6048   2008027627

Printed in the United States of America
12 11 10 09 08   10 9 8 7 6 5 4 3 2 1

To Raj Jandial and his family (Sonali, Uma, and Arjun)–both brother and friend, your lifelong support has made an indelible impact on my career and life.

Rahul Jandial

To my parents, Linda Page Hughes and John Richard Hughes, an exceedingly small return on their continued, colossal investment.

Samuel A. Hughes

To my stepfather, Robert Weiskopf, PhD, whose inquisitive mind, bright personality, and ceaseless energy are dearly missed by his friends, family, colleagues, and students.

Charles B. Newman

CONTENTS

Preface   ix

Part 1: The Healthy Brain and Skull   *1*

Questions 1–8 describe the function and anatomy of the brain and skull:
- What is the function of the skull?
- What is the surface anatomy of the brain?
- How are brain function and recovery different in children versus in adults?

Part 2: Head Trauma   *13*

Questions 9–22 cover the basics of head trauma and brain injury, such as causes, symptoms, and tests:
- What is head/brain injury?
- Why does the injured brain swell?
- How is brain injury evaluated in the hospital?

Part 3: Head Trauma in Children Versus Adults   *29*

Questions 23–26 address the anatomy of a child's skull compared to that of an adult, and how head trauma differs between them:
- What are the differences between a child's skull and an adult's skull?
- Do children recover better than adults after head trauma or brain injury?
- Can skull fractures expand in kids?

Part 4: Types of Head Trauma   *33*

Questions 27–36 explore different types of injury to the brain and skull:
- What is a scalp laceration?
- Which types of skull fractures need to be operated on?
- What is a subdural hematoma (SDH)?

Part 5: Coma   45

Questions 37–44 discuss altered mental status, loss of consciousness, and coma:
- What is the difference between altered mental status and loss of consciousness?
- What is diffuse axonal injury (DAI)?
- When does coma become brain death?

Part 6: Treating Head Trauma   53

Questions 45–54 cover different ways of treating head trauma, including medications and types of surgery:
- What medications can help relieve brain swelling?
- What surgery can help relieve brain swelling?
- What are the risks of brain surgery for head trauma and brain injury?

Part 7: The Head-Injured Patient in the Hospital   65

Questions 55–63 describe what patients with head injuries, from mild to severe, and their families can expect while they are in the hospital:
- Why do I have to stay in the hospital if I have only mild head injury?
- How is pain treated in patients with a head injury?
- Do patients with a concussion need to be kept awake for 24 hours after an injury?

Part 8: Persistent Vegetative States   73

Questions 64–73 describe what happens when a person is in a vegetative state or coma as a result of head trauma:
- What is a vegetative state?
- Are there any tests that can be done to determine if a person is in a coma or a PVS, or if he or she will ever wake up?
- What does it mean to withdraw care?

Part 9: Post-Concussive Syndrome   81

Questions 74–82 explore what happens during and after a concussion:
- What is a concussion?
- What causes post-concussive syndrome?
- When can I start playing sports or being active again?

Part 10: Long-Term Consequences of Head Injury   87

Questions 83–90 address possible issues that can arise following head trauma:
- What sort of neurological problems are expected following a brain injury?
- What kinds of cognitive problems can head injury cause?
- How much function will I regain?

Part 11: Rehabilitation after Head Trauma and Brain Injury   95

Questions 91–100 describe how the brain is able to recover and what a person with head injury can expect during the rehabilitation process:
- How long does it take to recover from a head injury?
- What kinds of problems can I expect during rehabilitation?
- Can severe head injury cause changes in personality?

Appendix   103

A list of resources and organizations that provide support to those affected by head trauma or brain injury.

Glossary   105

Index   111

The treatment of patients with traumatic brain injury remains one of the most challenging problems in modern medicine, both for clinicians and for the patients' friends, family members, and other loved ones. Although our fund of knowledge for providing care has increased in recent decades, even today the outcomes of these injuries can be disheartening due to the inherent fragility of the brain and its need for functional integrity in order to serve as the seat of an individual's mind and identity. The ongoing dialogue on this subject can be very difficult to understand, and it is for this reason that this text has been written as a resource for anyone involved in the care and rehabilitation of a person with a traumatic brain injury. To this end, the utmost effort has been made to provide the reader with a meaningful amount of current, critical information in a writing style that is comprehensible to a wide audience.

100 Questions & Answers About Head and Brain Injuries offers relevant background on normal brain anatomy along with its discussion of the various types of surgical and nonsurgical forms of head and brain injury. Further, significant attention has been given to the discussion both of prognosis and of rehabilitation, which remains a major factor in the ultimate maximal recovery of the head-injured patient. We hope that this text helps the reader navigate what is for most an unfamiliar and unwelcoming terrain.

Rahul Jandial, MD, PhD

PART ONE

The Healthy Brain and Skull

What is the function of the skull?

What is the anatomy of the skull?

How are brain function and recovery different in children versus in adults?

More . . .

Central nervous system (CNS)

Pertaining to the brain and spinal cord.

Cerebellum

Part of the brain located at the back of the head, under the cerebrum and in front of the brain stem. Controls balance and coordination, affecting movements of the same side of the body.

Ventricle

From Latin for "little belly," a ventricle is a fluid-filled space. The brain has four separate spaces within it called ventricles, all of which are filled with cerebrospinal fluid.

Fontanelles

Commonly called "soft spots," the fontanelles are the portions of the skull not yet ossified in infants; they usually fuse between the first and second years of life.

1. When do the brain and skull form?

The brain is part of the **central nervous system (CNS)** and begins to develop in the fetus from very early in pregnancy. At this point the brain is not fully formed, but more of a zone of tissue from which the brain will ultimately develop. This nervous system tissue arises from a layer of tissue in the embryo called the neuroectoderm. Throughout pregnancy the brain continues to develop and the structures of the brain take shape. These structures will be discussed in more detail elsewhere, but they include the brain lobes, **cerebellum**, brain fluid chambers (called **ventricles**), and brain arteries and veins. Amazingly, the brain continues to develop even after birth. The structures of the brain and the nervous system continue to mature throughout childhood and into young adulthood. One example of this ongoing process is how children become more coordinated in the first few years of life and learn to walk and talk. This progress occurs because the central nervous system, including the brain, continues to develop and strengthen in function after birth.

Like the brain, the skull continues to mature even after birth. As the bony plates of the skull grow together to form the completely enclosed skull, openings called **fontanelles**, commonly called "soft spots," remain. The fontanelles close by age two. The anterior fontanelle, the "soft spot" behind the forehead, is usually the last to close.

Although the brain matures after birth, most parts of the brain cannot regrow or regenerate if injured. Some organs, like the liver, can be significantly injured and still perform the function required by the body. The liver itself can even regenerate tissue obliterated by injury or disease. The brain is an organ quite different from the liver inasmuch as even microscopic areas of damage can leave the organ dysfunctional and its ability to regenerate is highly limited.

2. What is the function of the skull?

The rigid skull houses and protects the delicate brain. The interior of the skull develops in a shape that matches the shape of the brain and contains holes (called foramina, singular foramen) through which structures can enter (like arteries) or exit (like veins, the spine, and the **cranial nerves**) to serve the brain and facilitate its function.

3. What is the anatomy of the skull?

The skull is composed of various bony plates that ultimately grow into each other in a process called fusion and make a nearly complete bony enclosure (except for the foramina) (Figure 1). The frontal bone makes up the forehead, and after age seven it can have a bubble of air within it called a sinus. The bones in our temple region are called the temporal bones and are the thinnest bones in our skull, and the bones on the side of the skull are called the parietal bones. The bone in the back of the head is the occipital bone, and at the bottom is a large hole called the **foramen magnum**, through which the spinal cord passes.

The skull is further divided into internal regions by connective tissue called the **falx cerebri** ("the scythe of the brain") and the **tentorium cerebelli** ("the cerebellum's tent"). The falx splits the skull into left and right hemispheres and takes the shape of a "Mohawk" haircut inside the middle of the skull extending from the forehead to the back of the head. Like a tent under which the cerebellum takes cover, the tentorium extends from side to side with the cranial vault and splits the **occipital lobe** of the brain from the cerebellum. These structures are rigid enough to keep the brain from shifting within the skull under normal conditions, but they can also damage the brain by resisting it when it is shifted due to injury.

Cranial nerves

Nerves that arise from the base of the brain or the brain stem that provide sensory and motor functions to the eyes, nose, ears, tongue, and face.

Foramen magnum

The hole at the base of the skull through which the spinal cord emerges.

Falx cerebri

A fold of dura mater that divides the left and right cerebral hemispheres from one another.

Tentorium cerebelli

A fold of the dura that covers the cerebellum and divides it from the cerebrum; it has a hole in the middle of it through which the brain stem passes called the "incisura tentorii."

Occipital lobe

The area in the cerebral hemispheres that interprets visual images as well as the meaning of written words.

The Healthy Brain and Skull

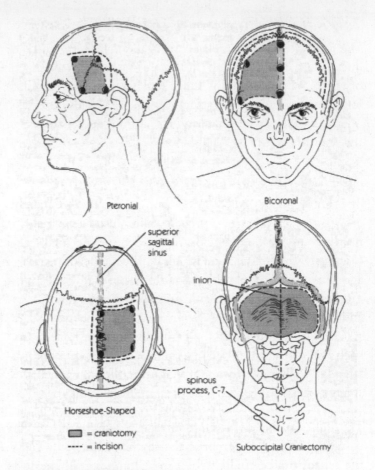

Pteronial

Bicoronal

superior
sagittal
sinus

inion

spinous
process, C-7

Horseshoe-Shaped

■ = craniotomy
---- = incision

Suboccipital Craniectomy

Figure 1. The skull's anatomy.

4. What is the surface anatomy of the brain?

Hemisphere

One of the two halves of the cerebrum or cerebellum.

Frontal lobe

The anterior (toward the face) area in the cerebral hemisphere involved in emotion, thought, reasoning, and behavior.

The surface of the brain has the characteristic cobblestone pattern with which we are all familiar. The hills and valleys along the brain's surface are called gyri and sulci, respectively. This shape increases the brain's surface area relative to its overall size. The brain is split into the left and right **hemispheres**. The falx is located within this cleft. The cerebellum (below the tentorium) also has its own left and right hemispheres joined by a midline tubular structure called the vermis, a Latin word meaning "worm."

The individual hemispheres are divided further into lobes. This separation is based on function and less easy to detect based only on surface anatomy. Both hemispheres have a **frontal lobe** (behind the frontal bone), a **temporal lobe** (mostly beneath the respective temporal bones), a **parietal lobe** (beneath the parietal bones), and an occipital lobe (beneath the occipital bones). The cerebellar lobes are also beneath the occipital bone and toward the back of the head where it connects to the neck.

The brain also has certain layers and compartments that provide organization to the way the brain is housed within the skull and become relevant when evaluating the location and type of brain hemorrhage in the setting of trauma. One way the layers can be conceptualized is by starting with the scalp and entering deeper inside to the skull, the surface of the brain, and, ultimately, the compartments of the brain itself.

Just underneath the scalp is the skull. Between the skull and the brain are three layers of tissue. The first is a connective tissue membrane called the **dura mater**, a sac-like covering of the brain. Accordingly, the space between the skull and the dura is called the epidural space, and the space between the dura and the brain is called the subdural space. Another membrane enters the surface of the brain and actually follows intimately through each hill and valley (gyrus and sulcus) of tissue on the surface of the brain. This layer is called the arachnoid and is very thin and delicate, like a cobweb. Finally, there is a membrane that clings tenaciously to the brain's surface and is nearly indistinguishable from the brain itself. This layer is called the pia.

The surface of the brain, called the **cortex**, is where the majority of the neurons live. Because of their color, this area is also called the gray matter. Deep within this layer is an area through which the neurons send their processes to the **brain stem** and spinal cord. This area is called white matter, because the insulation around the processes appears white

The Healthy Brain and Skull

Temporal lobe

The area in the cerebral hemispheres that contain both the auditory and visual pathways and the interpretation of sounds and spoken language for long-term memory.

Parietal lobe

The area in the cerebral hemispheres that controls sensory and motor information.

Dura mater

The outermost covering of the brain, a tough and fibrous membrane found immediately under the skull.

Cortex

The outer surface of the cerebral hemispheres; often called the gray matter.

Brain stem

The part of the central nervous system responsible for a number of "unconscious" activities, including breathing, heart rate, wakefulness, and sleep.

when analyzed by pathologists. Within the center of the brain are the ventricles that contain spinal fluid. Around and beneath these structures are a smaller number of neurons than on the outside layer. These neurons are clustered in specific structures that have to do with transmitting signals between the brain and body and are called the deep gray structures, or basal ganglia.

5. What are the different regions of the brain?

The brain regions include the lobes and hemispheres mentioned in Question 4, as well as other regions that are not visible on the surface of the brain and are critical to normal brain function (Figure 2 and Table 1).

Table 1. Functions of the different brain regions.

Frontal lobe	Responsible for complex thoughts, math, abstract thinking
Parietal lobe	Houses movement and sensation centers Responsible for 3-D processing
Temporal lobe	Responsible for language and memory
Occipital lobe	Responsible for vision
Cerebellum	Responsible for coordination Makes movements smooth
Brain stem	Responsible for movement and sensation Responsible for consciousness

The cortex of the brain is the outer surface of the brain. This surface is about half an inch thick and is made of the nuclei (the engines) of the brain cells, and when the brain is dissected the cortex has a unique gray color due to its housing the brain cell nuclei. Hence, the cortex is called gray matter. This gray matter (made up of brain cell nuclei) communicates with other parts of the brain via their axons (analogous to arms). The axons are white in color, and the region of the brain in which they are found is called white matter.

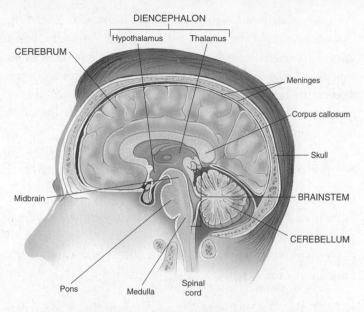

Figure 2. This image describes the major regions of the brain—the cerebrum, the cerebellum, and the brain stem.

Reproduced from Alters S, *Biology: Understanding Life*, Third Edition. © 2000 Jones and Bartlett Publishers, LLC. Sudbury, Massachusetts.

Beneath the surface of the brain is the subcortical region. The subcortical region functions as a relay station between the brain cells in the cortex and the brain stem and spinal cord. It also serves as a relay station and editor for information coming from the spinal cord and headed to the brain. Patients with movement disorders often have disease in the subcortical region. Damage to subcortical brain structure is debilitating not because of the loss of ability to move, but from the lack of proper coordination of movement. Subtle movements, especially complex tasks with our hands, are what enable us to live our daily lives. Altering these movements can make normal function difficult.

Another region of the brain is known as the brain stem. Using a mushroom as a visual example, the cap would be analogous to the brain and the stalk would be analogous to the brain

Consciousness

Emerging from a combination of a part of the brain stem that causes overall arousal and the function of both cerebral hemispheres, consciousness is the state of both awareness of the world and active volition in carrying out actions.

Neurological deficit

The partial or complete loss of muscle strength, sensation, or other brain functions; may be temporary or permanent.

Neurosurgeon

A surgical specialist whose area of concentration includes the management and treatment of acute intracranial and spinal injuries.

stem. The brain stem is the conduit for information heading from the brain to the spinal cord and vice versa. The brain stem also has smaller regions that are the origin of nerves that control the movements of the eyes, face, and structures in the throat. The brain stem also houses the areas responsible for **consciousness** and respiration and communicates impulses to the brain and spine.

6. Are some regions of the brain more essential for consciousness than others?

Absolutely. Consciousness—or, more simply, being awake—is something for which the brain is responsible. However, not all parts of the brain are necessary for consciousness and others are critically important.

Because the responsibility for consciousness is widely distributed with the brain, a single frontal lobe, occipital lobe, parietal lobe, or frontal lobe can be removed and will lead to **neurological deficits**, but with minimal change in consciousness. The brain stem, however, houses a structure called the reticular activating system, which is responsible for stimulating the brain to produce consciousness. For consciousness to be altered, therefore, it requires either global (or near global) brain injury—such as with general elevation of brain pressure or injury to both frontal lobes—or injury to the specific structure of the reticular activating system with the brain stem or its communication pathway with the brain. Even then, consciousness is a very complicated process and cannot be understood simply on mechanical terms. For the purpose of understanding the debilitation potentially associated with head injury, the particular brain regions injured are the major predictors of whether a person will lose the ability to be awake or will remain unconscious.

A **neurosurgeon** may elect to keep the patient in an unconscious state by giving strong sedative medicines in order to minimize brain swelling and prevent further brain injury and should not be confused with the ultimate potential for a person to recover brain function (such as consciousness). At a safe point the neurosurgeon will remove the sedative medicines, and as the body clears these drugs the person's full function and recovery potential can be evaluated.

Dennis's comments:

Though my TBI was contained to the right temporal region of my brain, since the global impact was so significant, it altered my consciousness so much so that I was comatose then semi-comatose for more than two weeks. But since my brain stem seemed to be unaffected save for a temporary elevation in brain pressure, as my injury healed and my brain stabilized I regained consciousness.

7. What is the function of the fluid compartments in the brain (ventricles)?

The brain is composed of tissue floating in brain fluid (called **cerebrospinal fluid**) and housed within the skull, and it also has central fluid chambers called ventricles. Ventricles are the source of the cerebrospinal fluid and can be found in both cerebral hemispheres (with different portions within the frontal, temporal, parietal, and occipital lobes) (Figure 3).

The ventricles are labeled as the **lateral ventricles** (one within each cerebral hemisphere), the **third ventricle** (at the brain's very center and connecting the two lateral ventricles), and the **fourth ventricle** (located behind the cerebellum). The cerebrospinal fluid is continuously generated within the ventricles, passes through the substance of the brain, exits near the brain stem, bathes the surface of the brain, and also provides the liquid environment in which the brain floats. The fluid is ultimately absorbed from the surface of the brain into the veins via structures called arachnoid granulations. The fluid chambers are fundamental to the care of the brain when related to brain/head injury, as will be discussed later.

Cerebrospinal fluid (CSF)

Produced by a portion of the brain called the choroid plexus as a filtrate of the blood, cerebrospinal fluid (also commonly called "spinal fluid") both mechanically buffers the brain from trauma and clears its metabolites; imbalance of its production, transmission, or reabsorption is called "hydrocephalus."

Lateral ventricles

The two elongated, curved openings in each cerebral hemisphere connecting with two slit-like openings in the center of the brain.

Third ventricle

A spinal fluid-filled space in the center of the brain in communication with the lateral ventricles.

Fourth ventricle

One of the spinal fluid pathways in the midline of the brain, between the brain stem and the cerebellum.

Hydrocephalus
The imbalance of the production, transmission, or reabsorption of cerebrospinal fluid; may occur in the context of acute injury due to the blockage of fluid flow from its point of production inside the brain to its point of absorption around the outside of the brain and spine.

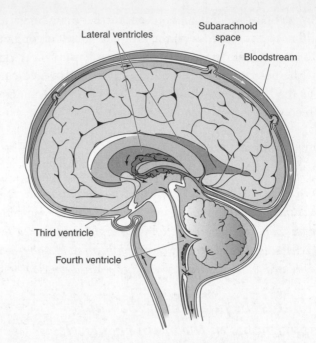

Figure 3. The major fluid spaces in the brain, called ventricles.

Adapted from the American Brain Tumor Association.

The ventricles in the brain are important sources of nourishment for the inner surfaces of the brain, and the chemical composition of the brain fluid is finely regulated. If the natural flow of the brain fluid from inside the brain to outside the brain is obstructed, brain fluid can build up inside the ventricles. This condition is called **hydrocephalus** and can lead to increased brain pressure, brain compression, and, if severe or if developed suddenly, death. If hydrocephalus occurs and the patient's mental status is deteriorating, a drainage catheter can be inserted into one of the ventricles to allow fluid removal and decompress the tense ventricles. This procedure is often applied to head injury as well, when it is necessary to minimize elevated brain pressure from brain swelling by removing brain fluid from the ventricles to make more room for the swollen brain. Brain fluid can also become infected. If infection occurs the physician will give the patient antibiotics.

If the natural flow of the brain fluid from inside the brain to outside the brain is obstructed, brain fluid can build up inside the ventricles.

On occasion the infection can arise from the presence of the above-mentioned brain catheter.

After brain surgery, brain fluid can sometimes leak from the skin incision, even when proper surgical technique and strategy are used. The chances of this drainage occurring are higher when the brain fluid is under pressure, as with hydrocephalus. Brain fluid leaks can be treated with additional sutures at the bedside or a small operation to reinforce the wound or divert some of the brain fluid from the spine.

8. How are brain function and recovery different in children versus in adults?

The brains of adults and children are both highly susceptible to injury, and their recovery depends directly on the type of injury and the area of the brain injured. As mentioned elsewhere, however, younger children have a developing brain, and some studies show that their brain is more "plastic," meaning that the function of an injured area can be recovered by improved function from another area of the brain. In adults, this plasticity is limited. Children who receive the proper medical/surgical/rehabilitative care, however, show an improved ability to recover when compared with adults with identical injuries. Brain injury is an extremely complicated and evolving field of study, though, and each injured patient has to be considered within the context of his injury by incorporating numerous factors that affect the ultimate recovery.

Brain injury is an extremely complicated and evolving field of study.

PART TWO

Head Trauma

What is head trauma?

What are the most common causes of head trauma?

What studies may be necessary in the hospital?

More . . .

9. What is head trauma?

Any and all trauma to the head is defined under the broad category of head trauma. A person can sustain head trauma and have no brain injury. Head trauma can include a concussion, a cut (laceration) in the scalp, a fracture of the skull, a gunshot wound, and all types of head/brain injuries. There are many ways to categorize head trauma. For example, injuries can be categorized by severity (mild to severe), by mechanism (penetrating or blunt), or by the presence or absence of direct exposure of the brain or its coverings to the outside world (open or closed). Head trauma is a field of medical, surgical, and scientific study on its own. Throughout the world head trauma is a significant cause of death, and those that survive can be quite debilitated. So, over the past several decades much interest and research has been directed toward minimizing the fatal and nonfatal consequences of head trauma. The overwhelming cause of concern with head trauma is injury to the brain.

10. What is head/brain injury?

Head/brain injury refers to when the brain itself is injured. This injury can be transient and not leave permanent damage, or it can be significant enough to cause coma or even brain death. The consequences of head/brain injury are directly related to the areas of the brain damaged and the amount of damage acquired. If a large area of the brain is injured, the resulting brain swelling that occurs afterward may secondarily damage areas of the brain that were not injured during the original trauma. The cycle can continue to where the brain pressures are so high that the entire brain dies—a condition known as brain death. If a small amount of the brain is injured, the risk of brain pressure is lower, but still present. If the small area of injured brain happens to be in an area where injury leads to few functional changes, the person can recover well. However, if a critical brain area suffers even a small amount of injury, the person may be devastated. As such, head injury and what that means for individual patients is highly dependent on many factors, and as such it poses a challenge to everyone involved in the patient's care, including the family.

The injury to the brain can be visible to the naked eye. Parts of the brain can be torn, cratered, hemorrhaged, or penetrated, as when something penetrates the skull and enters the brain or by an impact to the outside of the skull that is strong enough to make the brain bounce around inside the skull and smash into the inner surface of the skull. Injury to the brain can also occur at a microscopic level to the cells that make up the brain tissue. Cell function can be disrupted even though the brain may appear normal to the naked eye (such as during an autopsy evaluation) or to modern diagnostic imaging taken during the initial medical evaluation of a head trauma patient. The disruption to the cells can occur at an individual cellular level, to where the cells are less capable of conducting brain signals, or the cells can be disrupted in the way they connect to one another and thereby fail to pass along brain signals.

11. What are the most common causes of head trauma?

The causes of head injury vary with age, sex, geography, and lifestyle. There are, however, certain causes that overlap regardless of demographics. Using the mechanism of injury as a dividing point, we can review some of the causes of penetrating and blunt head trauma.

Gunshot wounds, stabbings, and piercing with tools (in an industrial work environment) or even writing instruments (mostly in children) are among the most common causes of penetrating head trauma. The famous case of Phineas Gage involved penetrating head trauma with a railroad spike that pierced the brain. Falls and motor vehicle accidents (cars, motorcycles, all-terrain vehicles) constitute the largest source of blunt head traumas. Helmets and helmet laws have significantly helped reduce head trauma. Being struck in the face or head or suddenly coming to a stop (as in a car accident) can lead to head trauma.

12. How does the skull protect against brain injury?

The skull provides a protective shell that encases the delicate brain. In blunt trauma, this shell absorbs the impact of any foreign object that would otherwise strike the brain directly. Specifically, in cases of high-energy impact in which the skull is fractured, because the conservation of energy allows impactive force to be used only once, the energy absorbed during fracture of the skull prevents the brain from receiving that force itself. Similarly, in cases of penetrating trauma, the skull also provides a barrier against foreign bodies penetrating directly into the brain.

13. How does the skull contribute to brain injury?

The skull is highly effective in protecting the brain by providing a rigid barrier to the outside world. The skull itself, however, can become a surface upon which the brain can strike. If the head is suddenly decelerated (as happens in a car accident or fall), the brain strikes the inside of the skull. Injury can occur both as it first strikes the inside surface of the skull (resulting in what is called a "coup" injury) and when it floats backward and strikes the opposite inner surface of the skull (in what is called a "counter-coup" injury), leading to minor or major head/brain injury depending on the forces involved. To protect against this injury, the brain is surrounded by cerebrospinal fluid and is essentially floating in this fluid within the skull. Unfortunately, this often isn't enough to prevent injury.

Dennis's comments:

In my case, my brain was not rattled within my skull; rather my skull was depressed into my brain. Indeed, the skull contributed much to the injury since bits of bone were driven into my brain, and caused high pressure on my brain and threw me into a coma for weeks. The neurosurgeons had to operate to lift the depressed bones off my brain, and allow it to decompress. My brain stabilized after surgery over a few weeks and I gradually regained consciousness.

14. What is the Monro-Kellie doctrine?

The Monro-Kellie doctrine states that because the skull is closed, the addition of "something" within the skull will necessarily lead to compression of the brain. The simplified model of the anatomy of the skull and brain shows the fundamental relationships between the skull's various contents. In it, the skull is thought of as a closed box of fixed volume. With this limited volume, under normal conditions, the skull must house the brain, the blood within the vessels that supply it, and the cerebrospinal fluid that suspends it. As such, under abnormal conditions such as in injury, it cannot expand as other space-occupying lesions are added in or around the brain. These space-occupying lesions can be tumors, hemorrhages, and/or retained cerebrospinal fluid (hydrocephalus). Thus, as the Monro-Kellie doctrine states, because the skull is closed, the introduction of anything else within it will lead to compression of the brain. At some point, the brain cannot accommodate any further compression and becomes injured, dysfunctional, and even smashed into other regions of the skull (a condition called **herniation**).

15. Why does the injured brain swell?

As seen in injuries to other parts of the body, swelling is a normal response to tissue damage. Because the brain is enclosed in the skull, brain swelling can lead to compression of normal parts of the brain, as well as of the nerves that originate from the brain. Brain swelling is a major threat to a patient's life after head injury, and much of the medical and surgical intervention used is to protect the uninjured brain from being injured by swollen brain. Also, brain swelling creates a vicious cycle of compression and swelling as a response to compression that can lead to something called diffuse **cerebral edema** (a condition in which the entire brain is swollen). Also, severe brain swelling can occur after minor injury to the brain; this

Herniation

The forced passage of one anatomical structure across a normal anatomical barrier, as in an abdominal hernia; herniation in the central nervous system can result in injury both to the structure forced across the barrier and the structure occupying the space into which it is forced.

Cerebral edema

Brain swelling that may result from increased vascular permeability or increased intraparenchymal particle content due to the failure of normal brain metabolism and the buildup of metabolic by-products.

head trauma

The treatment of brain swelling is complicated and involves several strategies.

exaggerated brain swelling is called malignant edema and is very difficult to manage medically or surgically.

Swelling of the brain happens for two main reasons. First, the cells that make up brain tissue can die and rupture. The contents from within the cells are spilled into the tissue of the brain, and the migration of the water that seeks to dilute them leads to brain edema. Second, the arteries of the brain have a unique barrier called the blood-brain barrier that limits what crosses from the blood to the brain. A head/brain injury can disrupt this barrier, leading to release of blood components (and, consequently, water) into the substance of the brain, once again leading to brain swelling. The former of these processes is sometimes called "cytotoxic" edema to refer to the cell death involved; the latter is sometimes called "vasogenic" edema to refer to the fact that it arises from the activity of the blood vessels themselves.

The treatment of brain swelling is complicated and involves several strategies. First, the patient can be placed on a **ventilator** and artificially made to breathe faster and deeper than usual. This hyperventilation can help reduce brain pressure and swelling. Second, medications can be used to help remove some of the fluid content from the brain tissue. Diuretics (water pills) such as mannitol can be extremely helpful for short periods of time. Steroids are not currently considered a medical option for treating brain swelling. Third, brain swelling can be improved with surgery.

Ventilator

A machine designed to support a patient's airway and provide needed oxygen.

If brain swelling is in a localized area (focal) of the brain (not diffuse), then one possibility for treatment is to remove some of the swollen brain with surgery. Of course, the patient must be able to tolerate the removal of these parts of the brain; for example, a person can tolerate loss of one frontal lobe, one occipital lobe, or part of the cerebellum.

16. What is the brain's natural buffering capacity against brain swelling?

The brain has some capacity for accommodating swelling or the addition of a space-occupying lesion, such as a tumor or hemorrhage. Initially the brain can expand into the space between itself and the skull. As swelling or compression increases, the brain can even collapse its fluid chambers (ventricles) to accommodate the mass effect. Next, venous blood can, to some degree, be squeezed from the brain's veins. Ultimately, the brain's natural buffering capacity is exhausted and significant injury occurs from the mass effect on the brain.

17. What is brain herniation?

When the brain's natural buffering is exhausted, mass effect pushes the brain into areas of lower pressure. This can happen as the whole brain undergoes generalized swelling after head/brain injury or even if a part of the brain (such as the temporal lobe) undergoes local swelling and mass effect. As described in the previous question, some of this movement is part of the brain's buffering capacity. These forces can, however, lead to brain herniation, when parts of the brain are essentially being pushed into an area where they do not belong. Specifically, the movement may entrap the moved brain and strangulate it from its blood supply, or the herniated brain may crush the brain or nerves meant to occupy the space it has invaded. Consequently, herniation is extremely dangerous and a complication of head/brain injury with mass effect (Figure 4).

There are four major types of herniation syndromes named descriptively for the area traversed during the herniation or the herniating structure: subfalcine herniation (herniation beneath the falx, from one hemisphere to the other), transtentorial herniation (herniation of the temporal lobe across the tentorium), central herniation (herniation of the brain stem directly downward from generalized mass effect from above), and tonsilar herniation (herniation of cerebellar tonsils into the foramen magnum) (Table 2).

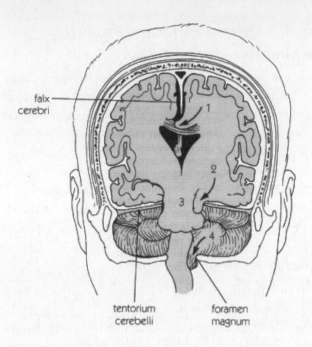

Figure 4. Four types of brain herniations: Subfalcine (1), Uncal (2), Central (3), Tonsillar (4).

Table 2. Brain herniation syndromes.

Subfalcine herniation	Herniation of the cingulate gyrus Usually well tolerated
Uncal herniation	Herniation of the uncus Most common type of herniation Shifted brain can compress nerves (resulting in pupil changes) and brain stem (resulting in coma and weakness)
Central herniation	Brain stem herniates downward Results in impaired consciousness and pupil changes
Tonsillar herniation	Part of the cerebellum called the tonsils herniates Compression on lower brain stem causes impaired consciousness and breathing irregularities

18. What are the signs and symptoms that suggest head trauma and brain injury?

Signs are findings that are noted on examination of the patient, and symptoms are what the patient complains about or describes (see Figure 5). Depending on the severity of the head trauma, patients can have a mild headache or be entirely unresponsive and comatose (see Table 5).

If the patient is conversant and oriented, a health care provider can obtain important information by interviewing the patient. Head trauma patients will describe a period of lost consciousness, headache, alteration in vision, light sensitivity, and even personality changes. If a seizure also occurred, they may also describe strange bodily sensations, weakness, and incontinence. Unfortunately, both head/brain trauma and seizure can cause transient amnesia, so some awake patients will be unable to describe their traumatic event.

On examination, head trauma patients often have cuts or bruises on their face and scalp swelling in the area of initial traumatic contact. A physical exam is performed that assesses the patient's ability to correctly state their name, location, and date. The person's strength and sensation in the face (determined by evaluating the 12 cranial nerves that arise from the brain), arms, and legs are also evaluated. If the person is confused, he or she is assessed for the ability to follow commands. If the patient is not awake, different provocative measures are taken to assess depth of coma, as this may reflect the severity of the injury. Reflexes such as pupillary activity, eyeblink, and cough can be elicited, as can response to tactile stimulation of the head, trunk, and limbs.

Depending on the severity of the head trauma, patients can have a mild headache or be entirely unresponsive and comatose.

Head Trauma

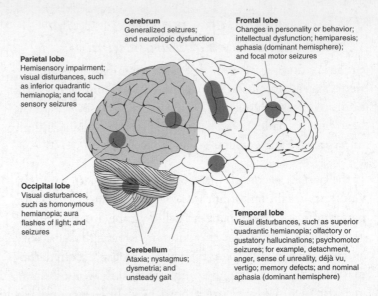

Cerebrum
Generalized seizures; and neurologic dysfunction

Frontal lobe
Changes in personality or behavior; intellectual dysfunction; hemiparesis; aphasia (dominant hemisphere); and focal motor seizures

Parietal lobe
Hemisensory impairment; visual disturbances, such as inferior quadrantic hemianopia; and focal sensory seizures

Occipital lobe
Visual disturbances, such as homonymous hemianopia; aura flashes of light; and seizures

Cerebellum
Ataxia; nystagmus; dysmetria; and unsteady gait

Temporal lobe
Visual disturbances, such as superior quadrantic hemianopia; olfactory or gustatory hallucinations; psychomotor seizures; for example, detachment, anger, sense of unreality, déjà vu, vertigo; memory defects; and nominal aphasia (dominant hemisphere)

Figure 5. The impairment in function one would have if particular regions of the brain were injured.

Adapted from *Coping with Neurological Disorders*, © 1982 Intermed Communications, Inc.

Table 3. Effects of injuring particular brain regions.

Frontal lobe (one side)	Injury to this lobe is usually well tolerated.
Frontal lobe (both sides)	Injury to this lobe results in significant debilitation.
	Also results in coma vigil, inability to initiate communication or interaction.
Parietal lobe	Injury to this lobe results in weakness and sensation loss on opposite side of body from site of injury.
Temporal lobe (left side)	Language area resides on the left side of the brain for majority of people.
	Injury to this lobe can lead to significant difficulties or inability to understand language (written or spoken words).
Temporal lobe (right side)	Injury to this lobe is usually well tolerated.
	There may be mild visual disturbances.

Table 3. *Continued*

Occipital lobe	Injury to this lobe results in visual field impairment.
Cerebellum	Injury to this lobe results in decreased balance.
	If there is brain stem compression, there will also be decreased level of consciousness.
	If injury results in obstruction of fourth ventricle, there will be acute hydrocephalus.
Brain stem	Injury to this site is highly variable based on location; results include but are not limited to cranial nerve deficits, hemiplegia, hemisensory loss.

19. How is head injury evaluated in the hospital?

In the hospital, if a patient is suspected to have head injury, several hospital teams will make a coordinated effort to evaluate the patient. Based on the signs and symptoms as ascertained by the history and physical exam, decisions are made on how rapidly the evaluation should take place.

Some patients are found unresponsive outside the hospital and brought to medical/surgical care by an ambulance or helicopter. Once in the hospital the emergency room doctors or trauma surgeons will be the first to evaluate the patient. For comatose patients, a ventilator is usually placed to help with breathing and imaging studies are immediately obtained. Depending on the findings of these original studies a decision is made about whether the patient has head injury and whether a neurosurgeon should be contacted. It is possible for someone to be neurologically altered or comatose and not have head injury, and the initial evaluation in the hospital helps clarify this.

For patients that are awake and conversant but have a history that may be consistent with head injury, imaging studies are performed on a less urgent basis and sometimes not at all. This initial evaluation is highly dependent on the story of the events leading to the presumed head injury and the physical examination performed by the clinician. Also, a decision is made whether to observe the patient in the hospital for a day or two, just in case a mild head injury worsens. This is particularly important for children, who are usually observed in the hospital.

20. What studies may be necessary in the hospital?

In the hospital or emergency room, a head injury patient will have blood drawn to determine if any drugs may be causing any altered mental status. Many substances both illicit and legal can lead to altered mental state, which can make evaluating head injury very difficult because it cannot be ascertained whether the mental changes are from injury, intoxication, or both. Also, the blood will be evaluated for coagulation abnormalities that could lead to or worsen any brain hemorrhage. These coagulation abnormalities can be medically created, such as when patients are taking blood thinners prescribed by their doctors. These abnormalities can also be simply previously undetected. Lastly, coagulation abnormalities can actually happen from release of substances from the injured brain. Regardless of the cause, if blood clots less well, then any brain injury associated with hemorrhage will be worse and lead to secondary damage to uninjured brain areas. If brain surgery is necessary, bleeding abnormalities need to be corrected prior to surgery and can delay life-saving surgical intervention.

Computed tomography (CT) scan

A scan produced by computer analysis of a long series of X-rays, a CT scan evaluates the relative densities of objects. In CT scans of the brain, the objects are usually compared to the normal brain.

While the laboratory evaluates the blood, a **computed tomography (CT) scan** of the brain is usually performed to obtain multiple detailed images of the brain, its fluid chambers, and the skull. Based on the physical exam, blood draw, and findings (if any) on CT scan, a patient's care plan is created.

21. What is the difference between a CT scan and an MRI scan?

Computed tomography (CT) and **magnetic resonance imaging (MRI) scans** are extremely useful in diagnosis of medical and surgical illnesses (Figure 6). In fact, their introduction has led to significantly improved diagnosis and much more focused surgical treatments. Computed tomography uses a complicated x-ray machine and a computer to create detailed images of the body's tissues and structure. This study usually takes about five to ten minutes, and most people are not too uncomfortable during the process.

An MRI scan is completely different from a CT scan in that it does not use x-rays and there is no risk of radiation. MRI uses magnets and radio waves to generate images. Some patients who have received certain types of surgical clips, metallic fragments, cardiac monitors, or pacemakers cannot receive this type of scan. During an MRI the patient will need to lie flat in a long narrow cylinder (the magnet) and part of the examination will involve loud clicking noises, which can take a total

Magnetic resonance imaging (MRI) scan

A scan produced by comparison of magnetic properties; various methods of analysis are used, resulting in different imaging appearances for objects that are magnetic or not; can demonstrate injuries to the brain not visible on CT scan.

Head Trauma

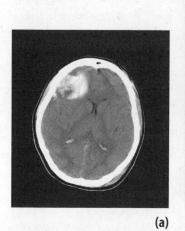 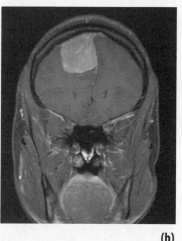

(a)   (b)

Figure 6. A CT scan (a) with brain hematoma (white area in frontal lobe) and an MRI scan (b) with contrast showing a brain tumor (bright white area).

of 20 minutes for the complete test. Some people find the narrow cylinder uncomfortable (those with difficulty with small spaces) and will need some mild sedation during the test. Some newer MRI scanners, known as "open air" scanners, are more spacious.

Both type of scans can be done with or without intravenous contrast. The contrast agents allow better differentiation of tissues and are used when the physician suspects a diagnosis that could be confirmed by performing a contrast-based study. Unlike for CT scans, the contrast agents used during an MRI are not made of iodine. There are fewer documented cases of reactions to MRI contrast, and it is considered to be safer than x-ray dyc.

When a patient has head injury the first and most helpful scan is the CT. This study can be performed quickly and provides information about skull fractures, brain **hematomas**, and compression of brain structures. Based on this study, physicians can make decisions about brain pressure treatment and whether brain surgery would be beneficial.

An MRI has little application for the immediate management of a patient with head injury. It provides greater tissue detail than a CT scan, but this increased information is useful when the patient is not in the critical phase of his or her care. MRI scans can be helpful in establishing the extent of brain injury.

Angela's comments:

This was a question that I always had before I sustained my TBI. I did not require immediate hospitalization, but when I went to my doctor's afterward, he recommended that I get an MRI done. Since my injury was not serious enough to require any immediate medical treatment, the MRI was the obvious choice since it is slower, but provides more detail. We were trying to determine the source of my symptoms at the time, and the extent of the TBI I had

Hematoma

A technical term for a blood clot; hematomas are often localized to the spaces either immediately inside the outer covering of the brain ("epidural hematoma") or beneath it ("subdural hematoma").

sustained. My doctor was very good at explaining the MRI and pointing out where the bruises were on my temporal lobes.

22. When is a brain surgeon (neurosurgeon) necessary?

After assessment by the emergency room or trauma team (depending on the patient's initial evaluation by triage staff), which generally includes a physical examination, blood draw, and CT scan, a decision is made whether the findings warrant consultation with a neurosurgeon. In general, any abnormal finding on the CT scan usually leads to consultation with a neurosurgeon, particularly if the scan shows any tumors, hemorrhages, or compressive lesions. On occasion, a person is comatose with a normal CT scan. In this setting as well a neurosurgeon will be consulted. Neurosurgeons are experts in the brain, skull, spine, and spinal cord, and accordingly they are the primary physician-surgeons that manage head trauma and brain injury in the initial phases of the injury. Clinical research into improving care of the head-injured patient has made significant progress benefiting patients who suffer head injury. These improvements include improving transport to the hospital, expediting the evaluation of head-injured patients, and creating teams of specialists in the hospital to provide coordinated and comprehensive care while the patient is in the intensive care unit. Also, neurosurgeons lead the scientific investigation into understanding the mechanisms behind head injury to come up with better treatments for the future.

Any abnormal finding on the CT scan usually leads to consultation with a neurosurgeon.

PART THREE

Head Trauma in Children versus Adults

What are the most common causes of
head trauma in kids?

Do children recover better than adults after
head trauma or brain injury?

Can skull fractures expand in kids?

More . . .

23. What are the differences between a child's skull and an adult's skull?

There are important differences between the skull of a child and that of an adult. A child up to the age of two or three has an incomplete skull, meaning that there are areas of "soft spots" or fontanelles that are not completely filled with bone. While these "soft spots" exist they provide advantages that the completely closed skull does not. First, they can bulge outward and provide increased buffering capacity for space-occupying lesions that may be added to the brain such as a blood clot (hematoma). So, in children, in addition to the ventricles, which provide some buffering capacity in adults, the fontanelles allow for some additional ability to accommodate mass effect. This bulging of the fontanelles also makes it easier to assess for increased brain pressure as part of the physical examination of the child. Lastly, the fontanelles make it easier and safer to drain the ventricles to decrease the brain's total pressure, as they can be easily accessed by a long needle rather than needing to drill a hole in the skull (as is necessary in adults to do the same procedure).

24. What are the most common causes of head trauma in kids?

Children are most commonly injured by falls from bicycles or skateboards (particularly if not helmeted). Also, some children suffer from falls from windows and can be severely injured. Also, motor vehicle accidents, whether children are inside the vehicle or struck by the vehicle, are causes of head trauma to children. Penetrating head trauma in children can also occur and includes gunshot wounds, stabbings, and piercing by sharp play objects. Helmets can significantly reduce head trauma and head/brain injury and should be used at all times when riding bicycles, skateboards, or inline skates.

25. Do children recover better than adults after head trauma or brain injury?

This question is difficult to answer because head trauma is a complicated injury and depends on many factors related to the injury as well as the care in the hospital. However, studies do show that children have slightly more ability to recover and, with the proper medical/surgical care and rehabilitation, can improve more than would be expected in adults with similar injuries. It is important to note, however, that the **prognosis** for every patient, whether child or adult, depends on the individual clinical case and is best estimated by the clinicians providing care for the head-injured patient.

26. Can skull fractures expand in kids?

In children, there is a risk that skull fractures (whether treated surgically or not) will expand as the child gets older. These skull fractures never heal, because a part of the membrane covering the brain gets stuck between the fracture edges and disrupts bone healing. The chances of this occurring and how it would be diagnosed and treated if it occurred would be discussed by the neurosurgeon involved in the child's care. Neurosurgeons look at specific criteria to determine if surgery is necessary.

Prognosis

The long-term outlook for survival and recovery based upon the patient's current status and the anticipated effect of available treatments.

Head Trauma in Children vs. Adults

PART FOUR

Types of Head Trauma

What is a skull fracture?

Which types of skull fractures need to be operated on?

Can the major arteries of the brain be injured with head trauma?

More . . .

27. What is a scalp laceration?

The scalp is the flesh that covers the skull and from which hair grows. During head trauma, the scalp can be bruised or cut just like any other skin surface on the body. The intact scalp over a skull fracture protects the brain; a cut over the fracture suggests a worse injury. This cut is called a scalp laceration. Patients with scalp lacerations are routinely evaluated for associated head injury, and it is one of the physical signs that raise concern for head/brain injury.

Patients with scalp lacerations are routinely evaluated for associated head injury.

Small scalp lacerations are usually washed with sterile irrigation and sutured closed in the emergency room or intensive care unit. If the scalp laceration is larger and associated with a skull fracture, a neurosurgeon may decide to repair the laceration in the operating room. This decision is made by the neurosurgeon and takes into consideration the injury as well as any other medical conditions the patient may have. Scalp sutures are typically removed one to two weeks after placement and can be done in the clinic with minimal discomfort.

28. What is a skull fracture?

A fracture is a break in the normal continuity of bone. A fracture can occur to any bone in the body, and the skull can be fractured as well (Figure 7). Skull fractures can be small and need no intervention or they can be large and need surgery. If a skull fracture occurs under a scalp laceration, the patient is at increased risk for infection.

The temporal bone is the thinnest bone in the skull and easiest to fracture. The pattern of the fracture can be linear (like the shape of a hair) and not change the general shape and relationship of the bone to other bones or the brain. The fracture also can be depressed, meaning a part of the bone is sunken in past the contour of the remaining skull. These fractures can injure the brain and be associated with brain hemorrhage. Also, depressed skull fractures can irritate the surface of the brain and become a source of seizures.

Types of Head Trauma

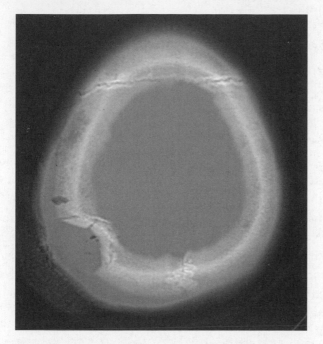

Figure 7. Depressed skull fracture: A CT scan (displaying images for evaluating bone) showing a depressed skull fracture.

Another fracture that can occur is a fracture of the frontal sinus. The frontal sinus is a bubble of air (and mucus) that is in the bone of the forehead behind the eyebrows. This sinus usually forms after age six or seven and can become fractured as well; some of these fractures will need to be treated with an operation.

Dennis's comments:

At the time, the neurosurgeons told my family that I had suffered a type of comminuted skull fracture called an opened complex depressed skull fracture. I later learned through research and consultation with physicians that this meant specifically that my skull was caved in against my brain, so much so that the skull fragments had torn my dura and my brain fluid was communicating with the external environment.

29. Which types of skull fractures need to be operated on?

Many skull fractures are linear and don't change the general shape of the skull. These linear fractures will heal in time (usually six weeks) and don't need any specific care.

However, some fractures will need an operation to realign the bone, remove any depressed bone fragments, and/or remove material (such as mucus with frontal sinus fractures, or debris with fractures associated with scalp lacerations) that can increase the chance of infection. Fractures that usually need to be operated on include, but are not limited to, the following: those with one or more significantly depressed bone fragments; those associated with an overlying, deep scalp laceration; those associated with brain hemorrhage; and fractures of the frontal sinus that lead to contact of sinus mucosa with the sterile brain.

Two types of skull fractures are unique because they require additional considerations. One type is a fracture of the cribriform plate. This bone is one of several bones that connect to make the flat surface upon which our frontal lobes sit. It is essentially behind the eyebrows and in the middle of the head. This bone has holes used for nerves to enter from the nose, and if a fracture occurs here, one potential consequence is brain fluid leaking out of the nose. Patients usually notice it dripping out of the nose when they lean forward (such as during shoelace tying) or they can taste the fluid when they lie back (the brain fluid is salty and drains down the throat). If this leaking doesn't stop on its own, then an operation may be necessary to either patch up the bone with tissue or divert the fluid out of the spine, so it has less chance to leak out. The other unique fracture is of the temporal bone. This bone houses the hearing apparatus, called the inner ear. On occasion fractures to the temporal bone can lead to hearing loss in the ear that is on the same side of the head as the fracture. If this happens, doctors responsible for the ear, nose, and throat (called ENT doctors) are asked for their input.

30. Can head trauma lead to brain hemorrhage?

Absolutely. The brain is a highly delicate structure with frag-ile blood vessels distributed throughout its structure. In fact, the brain receives a large amount of the total blood flow that leaves the heart. Accordingly, with head trauma, the brain can develop blood clots in various areas from a variety of mechanisms, including direct injury, shear forces, and striking the inner surface of the skull during rapid deceleration (such as happens during falls and/or motor vehicle accidents.) The location and type of clot are related to how a person tolerates the injury and what type of evaluation and intervention the patient may need. Some hemorrhages are well tolerated; oth-ers lead to immediate death. All brain hemorrhages should be evaluated by a neurosurgeon to determine the type of medi-cal/surgical/rehabilitative care the patient needs to maximize neurological recovery.

Some hemorrhages are well tolerated; others lead to immediate death.

31. What is an epidural hematoma?

The most superficial location where a brain hemorrhage can occur inside the skull is the epidural space. The epidural space is between the skull and the dura mater, the sac-like covering over the entire surface of the brain.

Because the skull has blood vessels within it that bleed when it is fractured, small epidural hematomas are found whenever a skull fracture occurs. The most severe hemorrhages in this area, however, typically occur in the temporal area, where the bone is thin. Also, the thin temporal bone has a blood vessel (called the middle meningeal artery) that courses intimately attached to the inner surface of the bone. When a fracture occurs in this bone the blood vessel is torn as well from direct injury, consequently pouring blood under high pressure into the space between the temporal bone and the dura mater. This type of hemorrhage can be rapidly lethal because the blood arises from a torn artery that continues to release blood under pressure (arteries carry blood under pressure) in the epidural space, even at the cost of smashing the underlying brain. The hemorrhage takes a classic shape on a CT scan, looking like a lentil bean or the biconvex lens of the eye (Figure 8).

The classic clinical picture of a temporal epidural hematoma includes some injury to the temple region of the head (such as being hit by a baseball) and a concomitant loss of consciousness. There is often a short period of recovered awareness (called the "lucid interval") until the brain is compressed to the point of causing coma.

An arterial epidural hematoma is a surgical emergency and needs to be operated on immediately. The operation consists of incising the scalp and making four holes in the bone over the affected area. The holes are connected and a square piece of bone is lifted, revealing the hematoma. The hematoma is evacuated and the torn artery is identified and controlled.

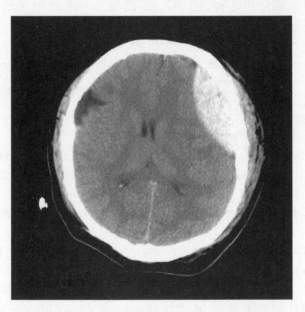

Figure 8. A CT scan with epidural hematoma (white "lens" shaped area).

Subsequently, the square piece of bone can be placed back on the skull and secured with little plates and screws. On occasion, a drain is left in place to remove residual blood and is removable in the hospital room without going back to the operating room. The scalp is closed with sutures. The patient is usually taken to the intensive care unit for postsurgical care of his or her head injury.

32. What is a subdural hematoma (SDH)?

The space beneath the dura is called the subdural space. This space, too, can be the location for brain hemorrhage after head trauma, an entity called a subdural hematoma (Figure 9). Subdural hematomas arise from the vessels that traverse the subdural space, which most often are the veins but can also be from small arteries on the surface of the brain.

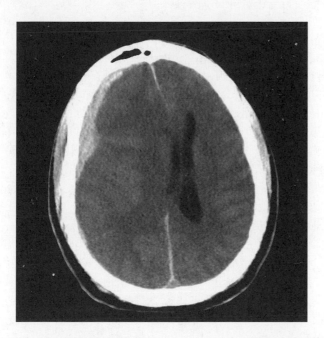

Figure 9.   A head CT, showing an acute right subdural hematoma with classic "crescent" appearance.

The blood can collect and cause a rapidly accumulating blood clot, like with epidural hematomas, and constitutes a surgical emergency. This type of subdural hematoma is called an acute subdural hematoma and requires emergent brain surgery by a neurosurgeon. The operation consists of incising the scalp and making one to four holes in the bone over the affected area. The holes are connected and a large piece of bone is lifted, and the dura is then incised, revealing the hematoma. The hematoma is removed and the torn vessel is identified and controlled. Subsequently, the dura is closed with sutures and the bone is placed back on the skull and secured with small plates and screws. On occasion a drain is left in place to drain residual blood and is removable in the hospital room without going back to the operating room. The scalp is closed with sutures. The patient is usually taken to the intensive care unit for postsurgical care of the head injury.

With subdural hematomas, the blood can also collect a little at a time, as the torn vein spills some blood and is compressed closed by the brain. This leads to something called a chronic subdural hematoma. A chronic subdural hematoma is usually better tolerated by the brain because the compressive effects accumulate over time. At some point, however, the size of the hematoma exceeds the brain's buffering capacity and it needs to be evacuated. The operation consists of making two holes in the skull over the chronic subdural hematoma, approximately the size of a nickel (2 cm in diameter). The dura is incised, and the subdural hematoma is washed out with irrigation into the two holes. This type of operation is possible only with chronic subdural hematomas, because blood that has accumulated over time (and hence called chronic) is liquefied enough by the body's breakdown of clot to be irrigated out. (In acute hemorrhages, the blood is clotted and can't be irrigated out, thus necessitating removal by a larger operation.) On occasion a drain is left in place to drain residual blood and is removable in the hospital room without going back to the operating room. The scalp is closed with sutures. The patient is usually taken to the intensive care unit for postsurgical care of the head injury.

33. What is intracerebral hematoma or contusion?

Epidural and subdural hematomas are on the surface of the brain. With head trauma, the actual substance of the brain can be bruised and vessels can tear, leading to a hematoma within the brain itself, called an intracerebral hematoma or contusion. The injury can occur for many reasons. One common cause is the brain running into the inner surface of the skull.

Intracerebral hematomas are diagnosed by CT scan and followed by repeated CT scans to detect changes in size. Often in the first few days after head trauma, intracerebral hematomas can increase in size (blossom) and lead to increased mass effect on the brain. If the mass effect is sufficient the patient can develop neurological changes and even develop brain herniation.

Depending on their size, location, and interval change on CT scans, intracerebral hematomas may need to be surgically evacuated by the neurosurgeon. The operation consists of incising the scalp and making one to four holes in the bone over the affected area. The holes are connected and a large piece of bone is lifted, the dura is then incised, and the brain is entered via a small corridor to locate the hematoma. The hematoma is evacuated and any bleeding vessels are controlled with delicate coagulation. Subsequently, the dura is closed with sutures and the bone is placed back on the skull and secured with small plates and screws. On occasion a drain is left in place to drain residual blood and is removable in the hospital room without going back to the operating room. The scalp is closed with sutures. The patient is usually taken to the intensive care unit for postsurgical care of the head injury. If there are many contusions and no particular clot to evacuate, the patient can be treated with a decompressive craniectomy.

34. What is intraventricular hemorrhage?

The brain is not a solid organ. It has within it a complex system of fluid chambers called ventricles. The ventricular system contains cerebrospinal fluid that fills the lateral ventricles (one on each cerebral hemisphere), the third ventricle (in the middle and connected to both lateral ventricles above as well as the fourth ventricle below), and the fourth ventricle.

With head trauma the brain hemorrhage can, on occasion, extend into the ventricles, although this situation is more often seen with hemorrhagic stroke. This hemorrhaging is of special concern because blood in the fluid chambers can clog the natural pathways in which the cerebrospinal fluid circulates. If this occurs, the cerebrospinal fluid builds up (because it continues to be formed but can't escape to the surface of the brain from where it is typically drained). This buildup of fluid within the brain is called hydrocephalus and can create significant mass effect as the ventricles expand and put pressure on the surrounding brain.

If hydrocephalus occurs, a catheter needs to be placed into the fluid chamber by the neurosurgeon to allow for necessary removal of excess cerebrospinal fluid. This catheter can be temporary if the patient ultimately can reabsorb all of the fluid created or, in some cases, will need to be converted to a permanent shunt underneath the skin to the belly. This is called a ventriculoperitoneal shunt.

In children with "soft spots" (fontanelles) the fluid can be drained by repeated needle puncture without having to place a catheter. However, if the child is ultimately unable to reabsorb all the cerebrospinal fluid the brain generates, a ventriculoperitoneal shunt may be necessary.

35. What is subarachnoid hemorrhage (SAH)?

A subarachnoid hemorrhage is located on the surface of the brain deep within both the dura and arachnoid. As such, it layers in a way other hemorrhages don't; it layers along any hill and valley (gyrus and sulcus) of the brain and even around the brain stem. This type of hemorrhage does occur after head trauma and usually is seen on the surface of the cerebral hemispheres. Subarachnoid hemorrhage usually doesn't require surgery and can be followed with CT scans while the patient is in the hospital.

SAH from trauma must be distinguished from SAH from a ruptured brain artery (**cerebral aneurysm**). This distinction, based mostly on the history of events provided by the patient, is an extremely important one. SAH from trauma is related to some sort of accident or injury. SAH from a brain aneurysm occurs spontaneously and typically is not associated with an accident or injury. Any suspicion of nontraumatic SAH will lead to intensive and sometimes invasive (cerebral angiogram) investigation into finding a blood vessel abnormality.

36. Can the major arteries of the brain be injured with head trauma?

The major arteries that supply the brain are the paired carotid and vertebral arteries. These arteries ultimately branch into fine arteries and supply the substance of the brain. With trauma the brain moves relative to the compartments created by the falx and tentorium. With this movement of the brain the vessels that are coursing through can be torn at the points where they enter the brain or traverse the falx and tentorium. This anchorage can lead to actual tearing with hemorrhage or the creation of a weakened artery (called a traumatic aneurysm). These traumatic aneurysms are prone to bleeding and need to be treated surgically.

Cerebral aneurysm

A pathological widening of a blood vessel that can be either local, like a blister or "berry" aneurysm, or gradual, called "fusiform." Aneurysms can be congenital or result from connective tissue disorders, infection in the cerebral vessels, or hypertension; these widenings of vessels are at increased risk of spontaneous hemorrhage, a potentially fatal event.

Treatment, if necessary, can consist of blood anticoagulation, endovascular stenting, and/or neurosurgery.

Also, the paired carotid and vertebral arteries that enter the brain from the neck must pass through canals in the base of the skull. With head trauma the vessels can develop tears on the inside surface of the vessel (lumen). These tears are called dissections and can lead to decreased blood flow through that vessel and ultimately to the brain. In some instances the injury to the arteries can be so severe that the entire vessel becomes clogged (occluded). These vascular injuries due to head trauma are extremely complicated and dangerous and require neurosurgical consultation along with those of other medical and surgical specialists in the hospital. Treatment, if necessary, can consist of blood anticoagulation, endovascular stenting, and/or neurosurgery.

PART FIVE

Coma

What is the difference between altered mental status
and loss of consciousness?

When does coma become brain death?

How is brain death diagnosed?

More . . .

37. What is the Glasgow Coma Scale (GCS)?

The **Glasgow Coma Scale (GCS)** was created to standardize the way clinicians categorize and describe a patient's clinical state after a head injury (Table 4). It looks at three main categories (V, verbal; M, motor; E, eye), and assigns points on a scale of one to six for each. The verbal category relates to the patient's ability to communicate, the motor category assesses the patient's ability to follow commands and move his or her limbs, and the eye category assesses the patient's ability to open his or her eyes.

Table 4. Glasgow Coma Scale (based on summation of highest points from each column).

Points	Best Eye Function	Best Verbal Response	Best Motor Response
6	-	-	Follows commands with face, arms, or legs
5	-	Oriented to name, place, and situation	Does not follow commands but exhibits purposeful movement
4	Opens eyes spontaneously	Appropriate speech but confused	Only withdraws to painful stimulus
3	Opens eyes to speech	Inappropriate speech but comprehensible words	Flexes (decorticate posturing) to painful stimulus
2	Opens eyes to pain	Sounds but no comprehensible words	Extends (decerebrate posturing) to painful stimulus
1	Does not open eyes to any stimulus	No sounds to any stimulus	No movement to any stimulus

This scale made a tremendous improvement in the way clinicians evaluated head injury and established a standard that can be used across countries and allows for a level comparison when people investigate treatment and prognosis for head injury (Table 5).

Table 5. Degrees of head injury.

Degree of Injury	GCS Score	Symptoms	Causes
Mild	13–15	• Headache (H/A) • Dizziness • Mild confusion	• Scalp bruise • Laceration
Moderate	9–12	• LOC • Seizure • Amnesia • Vomiting	• Depressed fracture • Basilar skull fracture • Intoxicated
Severe	8 or less	• Deteriorating level of consciousness	• Focal neurological deficit

38. What is the difference between altered mental status and loss of consciousness?

Loss of consciousness is what most people know to be when a person is "knocked out," like a boxer in a boxing match. This means that the person is not talking, his or her eyes are closed, and, usually, he or she is unable to stand up. Loss of consciousness is due to the brain not being in an awake state, but the person can be breathing and the heart can be beating. A person who experiences a period of loss of consciousness after head trauma needs to be evaluated by a doctor for head injury. People can lose consciousness for seconds or consciousness can be lost forever.

A person who experiences a period of loss of consciousness after head trauma needs to be evaluated by a doctor for head injury.

The term "altered mental status" is used to describe a person whose mental capacities are not normal, but the person is clearly awake and not "knocked out." These people can be awake yet confused, disoriented, or uninhibited. Altered mental states can occur from, among many other causes, drug use, fatigue, stress, dementia, general bodily illness, and head injury.

Any loss of consciousness or altered mental status in the setting of head trauma needs to be evaluated by a physician to exclude head injury that may require hospital observation or surgical intervention.

Dennis's comments:

When I first sustained my TBI, I had not been knocked out, or had a loss of consciousness. I was awake and talking to people, although I do not personally remember those moments; I was told that I was confused and disoriented, and really couldn't stand up off the ground. By the time the ambulance arrived, I had clearly lost consciousness, as, I suppose, my injury began to cause pressure to build up in my brain.

39. Are altered mental states and loss of consciousness always due to head injury?

No, there are many reasons that a person can have an altered mental status or loss of consciousness. Altered mental status can occur from use of drugs such as alcohol or other illicit drugs. It can also occur as a side effect of medicines given by a doctor. In fact, emotional stress, fatigue, and psychiatric disorders can frequently lead to altered mental states. These alterations can be mild, such as confusion about location or time, or more significant, as when the person is completely disoriented and cannot even communicate. Also, brain diseases other than head injury can lead to altered mental states, such as brain tumors, infections, and/or inflammatory diseases.

Brain diseases other than head injury can lead to altered mental states.

Loss of consciousness is also possible from non–head injury causes. When a person undergoes surgery, for example, the anesthesiologist uses medicines to create a controlled loss of consciousness. As with altered mental states, loss of consciousness can result from brain tumors, infections, and/or inflammatory diseases. Cardiac or cardiovascular problems can also cause acute losses of consciousness, as can metabolic disorders.

40. What is abulia or como vigil (coma vigilans)?

Abulia or como vigil is a condition in which a patient is entirely unable to interact with his or her environment. The patient is not comatose, however, because the eyes are open and sometimes even looking around. A patient with abulia doesn't initiate speech, responds very little to questioning, and is essentially "without motivation." This condition results from injury or disease to particular parts of the brain. The locations affected are usually both lower frontal lobes and, in particular, an area called the anterior perforated substance.

This state can also occur secondary to disease of the brain such as tumors, infections, and neurodegenerative diseases and has been reported as a complication of certain brain surgeries that involve risk to vessels that supply the anterior perforated substance. The recovery from como vigil is usually very minimal because the state is caused by injury to a specific brain region that if injured leads to permanent debilitation.

41. What is diffuse axonal injury (DAI)?

Diffuse axonal injury (DAI) is a type of head injury that leads to altered mental status, loss of consciousness, and even coma. This injury has to do with forces that cause rotational stress on the brain and lead to dyscoordination in the way the brain cells communicate with each other, particularly in the brain cells called axons—as the name of the injury suggests. Unlike in cases involving brain hemorrhages, CT scans of patients with DAI are often normal with no obvious lesion.

Based on the history of injury and the exam, DAI is a common cause of temporary coma in patients with head injury and no discernable hematomas or mass effect by CT scan; DAI can show up on MRI scans, however, that suggest this as the cause of coma in head injury. DAI can be so severe that patients do not recover and are permanently disabled.

42. When does coma become brain death?

When the brain loses function, the patient progresses through various stages of confusion, loss of consciousness, and coma, as graded by the Glasgow Coma Scale. Ultimately, if the brain is devoid of all function—and, usually, this is accompanied by a cessation of blood flow into the brain—the patient is diagnosed as brain dead. Brain death is very different from coma (which itself has various degrees). When a person is comatose, parts of the brain are injured (a condition that may be temporary or permanent), but other parts of the brain are functioning. When the entire brain stops functioning and the cells and tissues that make up the brain die, this is called brain death. It is not possible to recover brain function once brain death occurs. Patients do, however, have the potential to recover from coma, although the degree of potential depends on complicated factors related to age and type of brain disease.

Brain death is very different from coma.

43. How is brain death diagnosed?

The diagnosis of brain death involves physical examination, laboratory evaluation, and knowledge of the history of the injury or disease.

First, the patient's blood and urine need to be evaluated for drugs and medicines that can give the appearance of brain death, without the brain actually having completely died. Such drugs can include illicit drugs, alcohol, and medicines, such as paralytics, used by doctors. Also, the person must have a normal body temperature and normal blood oxygen/carbon dioxide. This is possible because the patients that are being evaluated for brain death are invariable invariably on breathing machines (ventilators), which can be managed to create the necessary laboratory parameters.

Second, the physician will perform a brain death physical examination. He or she will assess any movement in the arms or legs, as well as make a detailed examination of many functions of the cranial nerves that leave the brain stem and control unique functions and reflexes in the head and neck. For example, the physician will look at the function of eye pupils; check for the ability to cough, gag, and have spontaneous respirations; as well as look for other functions and reflexes.

If necessary, the physician can order tests that look at the actual blood flow to the brain; in brain death the brain receives no blood flow from the heart. The brain death evaluation usually requires two physicians, one of which must be either a neurologist (a doctor that treats brain disease with medicines only) or a neurosurgeon (a doctor that treats brain diseases with medicines and surgery). Other pertinent guidelines vary from state to state and nation to nation, and the physician providing care will discuss these guidelines, if necessary.

44. Does the heart stop beating after brain death?

Brain death doesn't require that the heart stop beating. This makes the concept of brain death difficult to understand when thinking in terms of whether the patient is still alive or dead. A patient is still technically alive if the heart is beating, even if there is brain death. However, shortly after brain death, even with modern ventilators and medicine, the heart often becomes unstable within 24 to 48 hours and the patient dies.

Before modern medicine a comatose patient usually couldn't breathe sufficiently and the whole disease process led to death of both the brain and heart. Currently, ventilators are used when a person becomes comatose and allow for respiration and sufficient oxygenation of the blood. Brain death doesn't lead to cardiac arrest immediately, and there is a period of time between brain death and cessation of heartbeat. During this time, a patient's family and/or legal guardian can decide to donate the bodily organs. Patients do not recover from brain death and will die within days, so organ donation from brain-dead patients is considered an ethical option. This option is presented to the family by a team separate from the doctors and nurses taking care of the patient. The decision is entirely up to the family and/or legal guardian, and no explanation needs to be given for deciding one way or another. Organ donation should never be pushed onto a grieving family; however, it is an option that some find helps bring meaning to a tragic situation.

PART SIX

Treating Head Trauma

How is brain swelling monitored?

What surgery can help relieve brain swelling?

What are the risks of brain surgery for
head trauma and brain injury?

More . . .

45. When does a person with head trauma need ventilator support?

A patient who has suffered head trauma may also have an associated head/brain injury. The extent of this injury determines how the patient is doing. Mild head injury may only leave the patient slightly confused, but wide awake and conversant. Severe head injury would leave the person unconscious and unable to breathe or keep his or her airway (trachea) open to allow successful air passage even if the person did have sufficient respiratory drive to take breaths. Moderate head injury usually falls somewhere in between.

For severe and moderate head injury, most patients will be placed on a ventilator to keep the airway open and protected, as well as to ensure adequate air is being sent to the lungs and brought out from the lungs. The ventilator also ensures that the blood receives enough oxygen (via the lungs) and that toxins from the blood (carbon dioxide) are adequately removed from the blood (via the lungs). This airway protection and breathing is very important not only for everyone, but particularly for patients with head injury.

Carbon dioxide that is not sufficiently removed from the patient's blood can lead to increased pressure in the brain by reflex dilation of the brain's blood vessels that increases their volume within the closed skull. Also, physicians will sometimes use the ventilator to remove more carbon dioxide from the blood than usual as a way to treat elevated brain pressure in patients with head injury by reflex constriction of the brain's blood vessels, decreasing their volume. Lastly, proper oxygen delivery to the blood by the lungs (and achieved by the help of a ventilator) is important to ensure that the cells and tissue in both the brain and body receive adequate amounts of oxygen to function properly.

A ventilator can be disconnected once the patient demonstrates the ability to protect the airway and breathe adequately.

If a patient cannot do this or becomes sicker, the ventilator is kept in place. Sometimes, especially when prolonged support is expected, the ventilator can be connected with a tube inserted through the front of the neck (called a tracheostomy) and not via a tube inserted through the mouth, as is usually done.

46. When does a patient need to have brain swelling monitored?

The window to how someone's brain is functioning is its performance during a physical examination. A patient's ability to talk or follow simple commands usually provides enough information for the physician to know if things are staying the same, getting better, or getting worse. If a person's exam changes for the worse, an emergent CT scan is performed to see what the reason is behind this decline.

For comatose patients who are not able to talk or follow commands, the **neurological examination** provides less insight into how their brains are functioning. This situation requires monitoring of the brain's pressure (called **intracranial pressure**, or ICP) with a device inserted into the skull and/or brain. The measurement of ICP serves as an indirect window into the condition of the brain. If ICP is elevated then the clinician can make medical and, if needed, surgical interventions to keep the ICP level under control. If ICP is elevated in a sustained manner, brain damage can occur from decreased blood flow to the brain itself.

47. How is brain swelling monitored?

Two main devices are used in the intensive care unit to monitor brain pressure (ICP) (Figure 10). The first is called a "bolt" and it essentially is the placement of a very small stylet into the surface of the brain (past the dura covering). This stylet is connected to a pressure transducer at the bedside and gives continuous measurement of the patient's ICP. The placement of this device requires a neurosurgeon and is done at

The window to how someone's brain is functioning is its performance during a physical examination.

Neurological examination

Part of the physical examination testing general intellectual function, speech, motor function, memory, sensation, reflexes, and cranial nerve functions.

Intracranial pressure (ICP)

The pressure within the fixed cranial vault that is produced by the relative volumes of brain, blood, cerebrospinal fluid, and "other" materials, such as tumor or infection; it can be measured with transcranial devices.

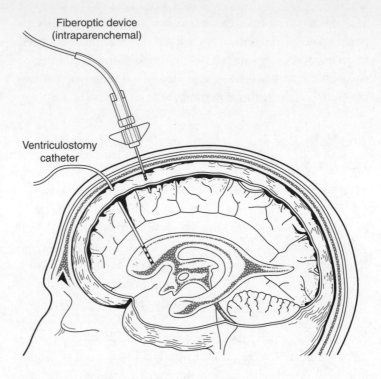

Fiberoptic device
(intraparenchemal)

Ventriculostomy
catheter

Figure 10. Devices for monitoring brain pressure.

the bedside with local anesthetic and a small drill. The scalp is incised (less than 1 cm or ¼ inch), and a drill is used to make a hole in the skull. Subsequently the stylet is introduced, secured, and connected to the transducer to give continuous ICP monitoring. The patient needs to be in the intensive care unit for the proper use of this device. Once the device is no longer needed, it is removed at the bedside, with placement of a single suture to close the scalp incision. The suture can be removed one to two weeks later by any nurse or physician. The procedure to place the "bolt" is a very safe procedure and rarely associated with complications.

The other option for monitoring ICP is called a ventricular drain. A ventricular drain not only offers continuous pressure monitoring (like the "bolt"), but because it is placed in the ventricular system, it also allows for removal of cerebrospinal fluid if ICP is elevated. This removal of ventricular fluid is one of the interventions that can reduce ICP and is considered a treatment for elevated ICP. The placement of this device requires a neurosurgeon and is done at the bedside with a local anesthetic and a small drill. The scalp is incised (approximately 2 cm or 1 inch), and a drill is used to make a hole in the skull. Subsequently, a catheter is inserted through the substance of the brain (usually the frontal lobe) until it enters the ventricular system. Once cerebrospinal fluid is seen leaving the catheter tip, the catheter is secured and connected to the transducer to give continuous ICP monitoring, as well as a drainage bag into which fluid can be released if needed. The patient needs to be in the intensive care unit for the proper use of this device, and once the device is not necessary it is removed at the bedside, with placement of a few sutures to close the scalp incision. The suture can be removed one to two weeks later by any nurse or physician. The procedure to place a ventricular catheter is a safe procedure, but complications of infection and brain hemorrhage during catheter insertion can occur. The neurosurgeon will discuss the risks, benefits, and alternatives prior to placement, if possible.

48. What medicines can help relieve brain swelling?

Brain swelling that is associated with head injury can be extremely dangerous for the brain cells and tissue. As such, the initial head injury can be made significantly worse by the elevated brain pressures that result in the days after the injury occurred, so patients with head injury are monitored in the hospital by their physical exam, CT scans, and devices that measure brain pressure.

The clinician has various strategies to control elevated ICP if it occurs. These range from simple raising of the head so the patient doesn't lie flat (this improves venous blood drainage and decreases ICP by decreasing the intracranial volume occupied by that blood) to medicines and devices, as well as neurosurgery. Of these various strategies, medical management of brain swelling falls under three approaches. First, medicines are given to sedate the patient. Second, medicines are given to remove some water from the swollen brain. Last, medicines are given to create a chemical state of coma, under which the brain activity is minimal as are the brain's metabolic needs.

Sedation is highly effective at reducing ICP because agitation and anxiety both lead to increased brain pressure. Thus, mild sedation is used if the patient's exam is to be followed; if the patient has an ICP monitor (bolt or ventricular catheter), stronger sedation can be used. Under the most dire conditions, paralytic agents can be added to deprive the patient of any possible pressure caused by muscle tension. Part of brain swelling is the release of water from blood vessels into brain tissue that shouldn't occur naturally. For this reason, medicines such as particular diuretics are used to help relieve brain pressure by removing water from the swollen brain. These medicines are dosed based on laboratory values that are simultaneously followed to ensure that the treatment is not leading to kidney damage. Also, intravenous sodium can be given to "dry out" the patient's tissues in a similar manner.

Sedation is highly effective at reducing ICP because agitation and anxiety both lead to increased brain pressure.

If a person has suffered severe head injury, one of the last treatment options is to place the patient in a coma induced by giving extremely strong sedatives called barbiturates. When all else has failed, this last effort aims to reduce the metabolic needs of the brain by making its activity significantly reduced. The thought is that with reduced demand from the brain cells and tissue, the swelling associated with head injury will lead to less permanent brain damage. This treatment is associated with many other risks, such as pneumonia, and is instituted only when most if not all other interventions to control brain pressure have been exhausted.

49. What surgery can help relieve brain swelling?

For patients whose brain swelling is uncontrollable by medications and ventricular drainage of cerebrospinal fluid, the neurosurgeon can perform a craniectomy. A craniectomy is brain surgery that involves removing large portions of the skull on the side of the brain. The objective is to increase the area in which the brain can expand when experiencing high brain pressures and ICP. With the removal of the fixed and rigid skull on the sides of the brain, the brain can expand further outward and is contained by the scalp. The scalp is more flexible and allows for some stretch as compared with the fixed and rigid skull.

This operation is usually performed either at immediate presentation or toward the later stages of severe head injury management; it is not used in routine management of head injury at most medical institutions. After a craniectomy, if the patient stabilizes and recovers to whatever degree from head/brain injury, ultimately the patient's own bone or a plastic shell modeled to the skull can be placed to cover the skull defects that were created. This is called cranioplasty.

50. Which types of head trauma need to receive operative treatment?

Head trauma that leads to certain fractures or hemorrhages is best managed by surgical intervention. Skull fractures that have significantly depressed bone, associated with hemorrhage, or involve frontal sinus exposure to the brain surface all require operative intervention by the neurosurgeon.

Also, epidural and subdural hematomas may require surgical evacuation. Intracerebral hemorrhages that cause mass effect may require surgical evacuation. In general, head injury that is from a hemorrhage leading to mass effect of change in neurological status of the patient is treated with operative intervention. After evacuation the patient will require medical management in the intensive care unit as well.

Also, elevated ICP that is not attributable to a specific brain hemorrhage warranting surgical evacuation and is uncontrollable with medical management can benefit from a craniectomy.

Angela's comments:

I suffered my head injury on the job. I was getting into an unfamiliar car and hit my head really hard on the door jamb. I knew something was wrong because it hurt even worse on the opposite side from where I actually hit my head. But there was no bleeding, no loss of consciousness, no obvious need to seek hospitalization, so I went home and rested. Three days later I realized that I almost went out of the house to go to work with shampoo still in my hair. That's when I knew I had to seek treatment. I ended up having bruises on my brain, but none of the indications for surgery: hemorrhage, skull fracture, or elevated pressure.

51. What are the risks of brain surgery for head trauma and brain injury?

The risks for any surgery include infection, bleeding, and death. The risk of infection is related to both the patient and type of surgery. Patients who are overweight or have diabetes are at increased risk of local and systemic infection after surgery. Also, operations of greater duration are associated with a greater risk of infection. To minimize risk of infection medical illnesses such as diabetes should be well controlled. Prior to the operation, antibiotics to cover bacteria on the skin are routinely given, and this protocol has been shown to decrease operative infections. If drains are left in place after the surgery, antibiotics are usually continued. Every operation has some amount of normal bleeding. However, the risk of excessive or uncontrollable bleeding depends on the nature of the operation and is greatest when major blood vessels are

The risk of infection is related to both the patient and type of surgery.

near or involved. Any underlying coagulation abnormalities that are not corrected prior to surgery will also significantly increase the risk of heavy bleeding.

The risk of infection is related to both the patient and type of surgery. The surgical risks in the setting of brain injury include these as well as other unique risks. Infection can happen with any surgery and is of minimal risk. However, if the patient has a penetrating injury or scalp laceration over the brain, the risks of infection are higher. If the brain or the cerebrospinal fluid becomes infected, long-term antibiotics are necessary and sometimes repeat surgery is necessary. Bleeding is always a risk with surgery, and the brain is a highly vascular organ. Removal of brain hemorrhages can also lead to the need to reevacuate the hemorrhage if it recollects after surgery. Any brain surgery can lead to brain damage, which can include permanent coma, paralysis, and even death. The risks, benefits, and alternatives will be discussed by the neurosurgeon. In many cases, the surgery is done emergently to save the patient's life, and it is the best option for survival.

52. Can surgery help uncontrollable whole-brain swelling?

At some point in the care of a patient with severe head injury medical treatment may not be able to maintain sufficiently low brain pressures (measured continuously in the intensive care unit). If this continues the patient will progress from severe coma to brain death, which usually happens as part of the brain herniates. Prior to herniation and after all medical management of head injury has been exhausted, some centers will offer an operation called "decompressive craniectomy." When a patient's condition is this poor, functional recovery is extremely unlikely, but not impossible. In this scenario and after discussion with the family, the patient will have two large circles of bone removed from each side of the skull. The bone removal would include parts of the frontal, parietal, and temporal bones. Since the scalp is elastic compared with the rigid skull bone, the brain now is given more room into which to swell, and thereby the total brain pressure can be reduced.

Sometimes during brain surgery for hematoma removal, if severe head injury is suspected based on the entire clinical scenario, the bone removed for access during brain surgery is left out, which can help provide more room to accommodate brain swelling.

Ultimately, if the patient survives the missing bone can be replaced by a plastic mold to improve the appearance.

53. Are drains used in the brain after surgery?

Yes, for many types of brain surgeries and especially after surgery to remove hematomas, many neurosurgeons prefer to leave a removable drainage tube in the operation site. This drain is tunneled underneath the scalp and connected to a device for fluid collection. If blood should re-collect after removal of the initially evacuated hematoma, the drain can serve as a conduit for the blood to leave the brain and allow the patient to avoid the need for another operation. Drains are not a replacement for a meticulous operation and do not always work; accordingly, patients are closely monitored in the intensive care unit after brain surgery. If a drain is used, at some point after the surgery, usually within a few days, the drain is removed at the bedside. Removal of the drain is reportedly only uncomfortable and minimally painful, and once it is removed, the small hole in the scalp where it was will be closed with a surgical staple or suture.

54. Do patients with head trauma need seizure medications?

Children and adults with head/brain injury have an increased risk of both acute seizure activity and, over the long term, the development of posttraumatic seizure disorder. If a patient has a seizure, then medications are always given to stop the seizure and then continued for various periods of time to prevent seizures from recurring.

Currently, there is insufficient evidence for or against the use of anti-seizure medications in head-injured patients who have not had a seizure. Clinically, these medications are still used as prophylaxis by many neurosurgeons. If judged to be appropriate in the specific circumstances of a given case, however, the evidence does suggest that anti-seizure medication should be used for only one or two weeks because these medications have side effects and do not appear to prevent the long-term development of posttraumatic seizure disorder. The medications taken to prevent seizures vary and have different side effects. Some seizure medications need to have their levels in the blood monitored and others do not.

PART SEVEN

The Head-Injured Patient in the Hospital

What can I expect to happen to my loved one in the intensive care unit?

What are the goals of hospitalization?

How is brain injury diagnosed?

More . . .

55. How are patients with head injuries monitored and assessed in the hospital?

If possible, a neurological examination should be performed at least once an hour by a medical professional, such as a doctor or a nurse. Sometimes it is not possible to assess a patient's neurological status either due to the severity of the injury or because of other injuries that require sedation as a part of treatment. In these cases physicians rely on CT scans and monitors (such as a ventriculostomy catheter or intracranial pressure monitor) to alert them when a change occurs. If a patient exhibits a change in neurological status (i.e., if he or she becomes less arousable or is not able to move part of the body that he or she was previously moving), then the physician will reassess the patient and the interventions being performed.

Monitoring of a patient's neurological status is the most important task during the care of the head-injured patient. However, the physician will also need to monitor all other parts of the body closely as well. Indeed, heart and lung function can be used to help control swelling in the brain, and lack of attention to these organs can actually exacerbate head injury. As such, severely head-injured patients are usually placed on a ventilator machine to monitor and control lung function. The heart is continuously monitored for abnormal heart rhythms, and the volume status of the circulation can be monitored by indwelling catheters in an artery. Tubes are also placed in the stomach and bladder for removal of excess secretions and delivery of drugs.

56. What can I expect to happen to my loved one in the intensive care unit?

Seeing a loved one in the intensive care unit can be a frightening and unsettling experience. Typically, a severely head-injured patient will require the highest level of medical care. The nurses in the intensive care unit are specially trained to care for critically ill patients and usually have to care for only one or two patients at a time. Neurosurgeons and trauma surgeons usually coordinate to care for patients with head injuries. Trauma centers typically have a neurosurgeon and a trauma surgeon available 24 hours a day. The machinery used to stabilize critically ill patients can be intimidating and confusing. Don't be afraid to ask questions of the doctors and nurses. A little understanding of the equipment used to care for your loved one might alleviate some of your anxiety. Access to the intensive care unit is extremely limited, with family and friends allowed to visit for short periods of time. During these visits, the nurses will help guide you to what can and can't be done. Young children are usually not allowed in the unit.

Neurosurgeons and trauma surgeons usually coordinate to care for patients with head injuries.

57. Why do I have to stay in the hospital if I have only mild head injury?

Head-injured patients who have neurological changes require hospitalization for their treatment. This can require a few days to a few months. Depending on the severity of injury and other medical factors (e.g., bleeding problems, major surgeries), a longer observation period may be required.

Even those with mild head injury should be observed in the hospital for 24 hours. Head injuries are unpredictable, and a patient's status can change rapidly. Ten to fifteen percent of the time, a minor brain injury will progress to a more serious, life-threatening condition. It is impossible to predict ahead of time who these at-risk patients are, which is why the physician will err on the side of caution: close observation is warranted. The initial observation period inside the hospital is a major part of the proper care of a mildly head-injured patient. Although you may "feel" normal, head injury can worsen. If it does, it usually occurs in the first few days, so being in the hospital with close monitoring could save your life.

58. What are the goals of hospitalization?

The primary goal of the hospitalization is to treat any immediate threat to life. In the case of brain or head injury, a patient may require cerebrospinal fluid diversion to relieve pressure inside the head or even emergency surgery. After stabilization, the goal is to prevent additional injury and put the body in the best condition possible to allow for maximal recovery.

The brain can continue to swell for several days after the initial injury, and if not treated the swelling can cause further damage to the brain. In the hospital, medical professionals monitor for signs of increasing swelling and will initiate treatment if appropriate. Patients who are on breathing machines, have urinary catheters, or have intravascular access devices in place for long periods of time are at increased risk for severe, life-threatening infections. It is important to protect these patients during this very vulnerable time.

59. How is pain treated in patients with a head injury?

Pain can be very challenging for medical professionals to help with. Very often, patients with significant head trauma have additional, painful injuries in other parts of the body. The most important piece of information that medical professionals use to determine the extent or current condition of a brain injury is the neurological exam. A critical component of the neurological exam is the level of consciousness, or how awake and interactive a patient is. All strong painkillers (i.e., anything more powerful than acetaminophen) have a sedative effect, and therefore they must be used sparingly in patients with head injuries.

Consider scenario in which a patient has a significant head injury and is given a large dose of narcotics to treat a fractured leg. If the patient becomes sleepy following the administration of this medicine, there is no way to know if this change in the level of consciousness is due to the medication or worsening of the head injury. The physician will need to perform additional interventions and possibly invasive interventions to definitively rule out life-threatening explanations for the new neurological status.

60. What is deep vein thrombosis?

Deep vein thrombosis (DVT) is usually caused by a lack of movement of the legs. Blood stagnates in the large veins of the legs and can form clots. These clots can be fatal if they break loose and travel to the lungs, a dreaded condition known as a pulmonary embolus (PE).

In the hospital, DVTs and PEs are a major cause of injury and are a major concern for any patient that is immobilized. Pneumatic compression stockings on the legs of an immobile patient may help stimulate the circulation of the blood in the legs to prevent a DVT. During standing and walking, it is thought that the legs keep the blood circulating by helping compress the leg veins and pushing the blood forward and back to the heart for reoxygenation. If someone is lying down for a long period of time the inactivity of the leg muscles can be compensated for with special socks that periodically squeeze the legs. This intervention for immobilized patients has significantly reduced the frequency of DVT and associated PEs. Another intervention is the use of low-dose blood-thinning agents. These agents are typically given twice daily and are short acting. Blood-thinning medications or surgically placed filters can also be used to prevent or treat DVTs and PEs. If surgery is necessary these blood thinners can be turned off and coagulation normalized. The combination of leg squeezers and blood-thinning medicines has decreased the risk of DVT for hospitalized patients. Occasionally, patients can not be treated with blood-thinning agents and need protection from the risks of DVT formation, specifically the dislodging of the DVT clot called pulmonary embolism. In this scenario, a filter can be inserted into the major vein that drains the blood from the legs and pelvis called the inferior

Deep vein thrombosis (DVT)

Clotting that can occur within the deep veins of the body, especially when someone is immobilized or more prone to coagulation by systemic inflammation.

vena cava. This vessel would be the final path in which a dislodged DVT clot would travel before getting to the heart. A filter in the inferior vena cava can be inserted by a small needle inserted in the inguinal area, and when properly placed serves as a net to catch any DVTs that may be dislodged.

61. Can brain injuries cause fever?

A high fever in the intensive care unit is frequently an indicator of a severe infection, but it can also be a result of brain damage. An area of the brain known as the hypothalamus functions as the body's thermostat. Injuries to the hypothalamus can result in an impairment of the body's ability to regulate its own temperature. An elevated temperature is the body's response to an infection or dysregulation of the hypothalamus. Regardless, severely elevated temperatures (greater than 103° Fahrenheit) can lead to brain damage and need to be controlled. To do this, interventions such as a cooling blanket or ice packs can be used to prevent the body temperature from becoming dangerously high. Preventing fever is an important part of the patient's total care in the hospital and intensive care unit. In the long term, patients may experience wild swings in body temperature due to the damage to the hypothalamus, which may manifest as shaking spells or excessive sweating.

Preventing fever is an important part of the patient's total care in the hospital and intensive care unit.

62. How is brain injury diagnosed?

A neurological exam is usually the best way to detect and diagnose brain injury. Sometimes, in the setting of severe brain trauma and coma, a neurological exam is difficult to perform. Gross damage to the brain, such as hematomas, bleeding, or swelling, is usually detectable on brain imaging, such as CT or MRI. Microscopic injury, as in the case of diffuse axonal injury, is not detectable on imaging studies. In these cases, the diagnosis is made by the history of the trauma (e.g., a sharp blow to the head, sudden acceleration/deceleration) or the symptoms reported by the patient (alteration of consciousness, headaches, dizziness, confusion, memory problems, etc.).

Ultimately, the diagnosis is made by physicians and incorporates all aspects of a patient evaluation. Beginning with a detailed history from the patient, or others if the patient is unresponsive, head injury is suspected based on the sequence of events. Next, a physical examination is performed and more details are incorporated. Examination of the skin, skull, eyes, pupils, and mental status can provide critical information toward a diagnosis.

63. Do patients with a concussion need to be kept awake for 24 hours after an injury?

There is no medical reason to keep a patient with a concussion or mild traumatic brain injury awake for 24 hours. This recommendation is outdated and appears to be based on the belief that a person with a concussion might slip into a coma and never wake up if allowed to sleep during the first 24 hours after an injury. However, a person with a concussion should not be allowed to sleep indefinitely. It is advisable for people sent home with mild head injury to be awakened.

An individual who is unconscious for more than five minutes, has persistent amnesia, or is otherwise behaving abnormally should be evaluated by a medical professional promptly.

It is advisable for people sent home with mild head injury to be awakened.

PART EIGHT

Persistent Vegetative States

What is a coma?

Can a person in a coma move?

Is there any treatment for coma or
persistent vegetative states?

More . . .

64. What is a coma?

Coma is a state in which a patient does not interact with the outside world. It is characterized by unconsciousness, unresponsiveness, and unarousability. Patients in a coma do not have sleep/wake cycles and do not respond to external stimuli, like pain or light. Coma is caused by severe brain trauma, either to the cerebral hemispheres or to the brain stem. Coma typically lasts only a few weeks, with patients progressing either to death or to a vegetative state.

The Glasgow Coma Scale (GCS) defines various degrees of coma. As a patient becomes more comatose, he or she also becomes less responsive, less able or unable to talk, and less able or unable to open the eyes. Based on these assessments the degree of coma is established. At some point, comatose patients cannot successfully breathe independently (from failure to keep their airways open or from depressed or absent breaths) and need to be placed on a ventilator. Also, the worse the degree of coma secondary to head injury, the less likely a full recovery.

65. What is a vegetative state?

Patients in a vegetative state, as in a coma, do not interact with their surroundings, but with some important differences. Patients in a vegetative state display sleep/wake cycles, may move their extremities spontaneously, or demonstrate primitive reflexes. The diagnosis of a true persistent vegetative state is increasingly rare, probably because of improved techniques for assessing severely impaired patients and because it is possible to keep survivors alive longer. Many vegetative survivors will progress to have some minimal amount of responsiveness over time. Patients in a vegetative state may or may not have their eyes open and usually can breathe for themselves. Although having open eyes is associated with a less severe coma, it doesn't by itself mean that the person is able to interact with the environment. So, a vegetative state is thought to be a condition in which the brain is able to perform basic bodily functions like breathing but still unable to respond and interact with the environment in a meaningful way. Family members of people in vegetative states may dispute whether their loved one is interacting in a "meaningful" way, and ultimately the decisions about quality of life for the patient and the family is theirs. Physicians provide information about what it medically means to be a vegetative survivor, and this information is incorporated by the family and loved ones into their decisions. Medically, although a vegetative state is not coma, this doesn't mean that it can be viewed as a transition from coma to full recovery. In fact, an overwhelming majority of vegetative survivors never become independent or even functional.

66. What is a minimally interactive state?

A minimally interactive or minimally conscious state is distinct from a comatose or vegetative state. A minimally interactive survivor displays behavior that is thought to be deliberate, cognitively mediated consistently enough for clinicians to be able to distinguish the behavior from reflexive responses. Patients in a minimally interactive state generally have a more favorable prognosis than those in a vegetative state. New therapies for patients in minimally interactive states, including drug therapy and even brain surgery, are being developed and may someday lead to effective treatments for this condition. Media stories of people "waking up from coma decades later" usually refer to people who were in a minimally interactive state. Describing these patients as having "awakened from coma" is very misleading, because vegetative survivors are in a different category than patients in a minimally interactive state.

Patients in a minimally interactive state generally have a more favorable prognosis than those in a vegetative state.

67. Can a person in a coma move?

Patients in a coma or a minimally interactive state can and frequently do display some movement of their extremities. This movement can be either spontaneous or in response to some sort of external stimulus (a doctor's examination or a loved one's hand squeeze). It can be very difficult to differentiate voluntary from involuntary movement, directed by the cerebral hemispheres from brain stem and spinal cord reflexes, particularly for untrained individuals. Primitive reflexes that are vestiges from our primate ancestors can become unmasked in the setting of brain injury, such as a hand grasp when the palm is stimulated. It can be challenging for physicians and family members alike to determine what the significance of an observed movement is, so be patient and ask questions.

68. Can a person in a vegetative state ever wake up?

Isolated case reports in medical literature do describe the phenomenon of a person in a persistent vegetative state (PVS) regaining the ability to interact with their surroundings, but these events are extremely rare, probably occurring with a frequency of less than one in a million.

69. Can a person in a PVS hear me?

Whether or not a person in a PVS can hear or understand language is an area of ongoing debate and research. There are isolated case reports of individuals in a PVS who demonstrate activity in part of the brain responsible for language processing on an experimental type of scanner. It is not known what the significance of this information is. Because individuals in a PVS cannot, by definition, interact with their environment, we have no way of determining whether or not this activity that we see on the brain scan is equivalent to hearing or understanding language.

When we think of a person hearing us, many parts of the brain are involved and many high-level functions and associations are invoked.

70. Is there any treatment for coma or persistent vegetative states?

Once the patient is out of immediate danger and has been stabilized from the condition that led to the persistent vegetative state, the medical care team will focus on preventing any further injury to the patient. This typically includes preventing infections and maintaining the survivor's physical state as much as possible, usually by preventing pneumonia and pressure ulcers (also known as bed sores) and maintaining adequate nutrition. **Physical therapy** is sometimes employed to prevent permanent muscular contractions (called contractures) that can lead to permanent orthopedic deformities that would limit functional recovery should the survivor emerge from the coma.

Experimental therapies such as deep brain stimulation (delivering controlled, mild electrical stimuli to deep areas of the brain) or drug therapy have been tried to induce neurological recovery, but conclusive evidence and guidelines for these practices have not been demonstrated as of yet.

71. Are there any tests that can be done to determine if a person is in a coma or a PVS, or if he or she will ever wake up?

Clinical observation is the best way to determine the extent of brain damage. A health care provider has to examine and observe the patient for a long period of time, sometimes weeks, to make the diagnosis. These professionals are trained to watch for subtle signs of higher cortical function. Different tests have been tried in an effort to obtain objective information about a patient's brain function. Such tests as glucose metabolism, **electroencephalograms (EEG)**, CT scans, **positron emission tomography (PET) scans**, and functional magnetic resonance imaging (fMRI) scans have all been used to increase our understanding of coma and PVS, but none

Persistent Vegetative States

Physical therapy

Therapy aimed at recovery from weakness, loss of coordination, or limited endurance.

Electroencephalogram (EEG)

An EEG measures the electrical activity of the brain; it can be used to detect the presence or absence (for example, in brain death) of normal electrical activity or to detect the abnormal activity of seizure.

Positron emission tomography (PET) scan

A nuclear medicine study that uses the detection of radio-labeled metabolic by-products; it is often used to detect normal or abnormal metabolism as is found in the context of injury and neoplasm.

has reliably produced information that can be used to make diagnostic or prognostic conclusions.

72. Can a brain-dead person move?

The concept of brain death is very difficult to understand. When a person is brain dead, the tissue making up the brain has died. However, the patient's body can be maintained for a few days by artificially filling the lungs with air via a ventilator. The heart continues to beat, blood is circulated by the heart, and the skin is warm. Regardless, the fate of this person is decided. A brain-dead patient can never recover and the body will shut down within a few days. During this time there is a window in which organ donation can occur.

A brain-dead person's body is not connected to the brain, and the arms and legs cannot move. There is one exception: the spinal cord may still maintain its reflexive connections to the arms or legs, so on occasion some small twitches may occur. This activity is completely consistent with brain death and doesn't mean that the brain is still alive or connected to the body. This extremely complicated process is one that will never entirely make sense, and the trust in and relationship with your doctor and nurses will help guide you to make the right decisions for your loved one.

73. What does it mean to withdraw care?

Withdrawing care generally means withholding invasive interventions that are designed to prolong life or treat a medical condition. If the difficult decision to withdraw care on a loved one is reached, the focus of medical therapy switches from cure and treatment to comfort and palliation. This course of action is usually reserved for cases where medical intervention is deemed to be futile, either at the request of the family or, more rarely, at the consensus of the health care team. If the extent of the injury is too severe to allow for meaningful recovery or if death is imminent and unavoidable, withdrawing care can sometimes be the humane course of action. For example, instead of administering powerful drugs to treat brain swelling or low blood pressure, the health care team might provide pain-killing medications to ensure that the patient is comfortable while he or she succumbs to the injury or illness.

A severely head-injured patient in the hospital is usually placed on a ventilator for respiratory support. If a decision is made to withdraw care, by the appropriate family member or whoever has durable power of attorney to make decisions on behalf of the incapacitated patient, the usual care withdrawn is removal from ventilator support. Essentially the breathing tube from which the ventilator provides air is removed and the patient is allowed to breathe on his or her own. Usually, if the recovery potential of a patient is limited enough to consider withdrawal of care, the person will not breathe sufficiently or even at all, so withdrawal of ventilator support will lead to inadequate oxygenation of the blood, which will lead to cessation of the heartbeat.

How quickly a person will die after withdrawal of care is a complicated question to answer. Generally the more comatose a person is, the more rapidly he or she will succumb when care is withdrawn. On occasion, withdrawal of care of a comatose patient thought not to have recovery potential will not lead to the patient's death. Sometimes patients will remain in persistent vegetative states. Family and loved ones must be educated about this possibility by the doctors and nurses involved in this end-of-life process.

Withdrawing care is not **euthanasia**, which is illegal in the United States. Euthanasia entails giving a terminally ill patient an intervention (usually drugs) that leads to cessation of the heartbeat (cardiac arrest). Withdrawing care does not entail giving any drugs that lead to death. However, medications to make the patient comfortable can be given for palliation.

Euthanasia

From a Greek term meaning 'dying well,' euthanasia is currently used to describe a set of practices that occupy a difficult medico-legal position and, ideally, produce a gentle and easy death in those who are deathly ill or debilitated without hope of recovery.

PART NINE

Post-Concussive Syndrome

What is a concussion

Who is at risk for traumatic brain injury?

How common is post-concussive syndrome?

More . . .

74. What is a concussion?

A concussion is a temporary, trauma-induced alteration in mental status. Some of the symptoms commonly associated with a concussion are confusion, amnesia, and sometimes a brief loss of consciousness, but a loss of consciousness is not required to be diagnosed with concussion. However, everyone who loses consciousness and regains it has had a concussion.

A complete loss of consciousness does not always occur with a concussion.

A complete loss of consciousness does not always occur with a concussion. In fact, a seemingly minor trauma to the head can cause lasting mental or physical injury, sometimes resulting in death.

Concussions are classified by severity, falling into one of three categories:

Grade I: No loss of consciousness, transient confusion. Mental status abnormalities resolve in less than 15 minutes.

Grade II: No loss of consciousness. Mental status abnormalities last more than 15 minutes.

Grade III: Any loss of consciousness.

75. Who is at risk for traumatic brain injury (TBI)?

Men are about 1.5 times as likely as women to suffer from a traumatic brain injury. The two highest-risk age groups are 0- to 4-year-olds and 15- to 19-year-olds. The leading causes of TBI are falls, motor vehicle accidents, inadvertent blows to the head, and assault.

People in certain military occupations (such as paratroopers) are at increased risk of sustaining a TBI, and African Americans have the highest rate of death from TBI. Athletes involved in contact sports, particularly football, martial arts/ boxing, hockey, and wrestling are more likely to sustain TBI.

Recently, risk of TBI from soccer has been recognized, particularly for women.

76. What is post-concussive syndrome?

Understanding of the effects of head trauma, particularly mild head injuries, is evolving and is the subject of ongoing research. Many patients, particularly younger patients, have persistent complaints after sustaining mild head injury, but they also have larger reserves and may recover easier and quicker than older patients. The diagnostic criteria for post-concussive syndrome are a history of traumatic brain injury and three of the following symptoms: (1) headache, (2) dizziness, (3) fatigue, (4) irritability, (5) insomnia, (6) concentration difficulty, (7) memory difficulty, or (8) intolerance of stress, emotion, or alcohol. Some patients may even experience loss of smell or taste, which may or may not be permanent. Historically, the severity of the head injury was thought to be primarily related to loss of consciousness. We now know that even mild injuries, particularly from repeated low-level impact, can result in serious, even permanent cognitive deficits, especially if a subsequent injury occurs within six months of the initial one.

The symptoms for PCS are similar to many other medical and psychological problems (e.g., depression, hypothyroidism, anxiety), so patients suspected of suffering from PCS should be evaluated by an appropriately trained medical professional. The psychological symptoms are more often found in patients who function at a (high) professional level and experience a reduction thereof.

Many patients, particularly younger patients, have persistent complaints after sustaining mild head injury.

77. What causes post-concussive syndrome?

There are two main contributing factors to post-concussive syndrome: microscopic brain damage and psychological factors. The relative contribution of these two components is not known definitively, and there is considerable debate in the medical community about this subject. Before the advent of sophisticated imaging technologies such as MRI, it was widely believed that the primary cause of post-concussive syndrome was psychological. Research has now demonstrated that microscopic and electrical changes can occur following even minor brain trauma. The recovery from these symptoms can largely be affected by cognitive therapy, the age of the patient, and his or her compliance with this training.

The real answer is likely that a combination of both physiological (i.e., true structural changes) and psychological changes contribute to post-concussive syndrome. Interestingly, post-concussive syndrome is more common in people who had preexisting psychological disturbances (e.g., anxiety or depression) prior to their trauma.

78. How common is post-concussive syndrome?

Some studies place the incidence of PCS as high as 50% following any sort of concussion. PCS is more common in women than in men, and people over the age of 55 are more likely to have persistent symptoms. There does not appear to be a predilection for age in PCS, but because the epidemiology for PCS mirrors that of head trauma, PCS is more frequently seen in children and young adults.

79. Why do patients feel nauseated after a concussion?

The reason for post-concussive nausea is not known. Suffering any sort of trauma activates the sympathetic branch of the autonomic nervous system, resulting in the release of powerful neurotransmitters like epinephrine (also known as adrenaline). Epinephrine is responsible for the effects of the fight-or-flight stress response (racing heart, pupillary dilation, sweating, clammy skin, nausea). Some researchers believe that this nausea is a result of an imbalance of the autonomic nervous system as a result of brain trauma. Others believe that it is direct trauma to the nausea center of the brain, the area postrema. The area postrema is a section of the brain located just above the junction of the brain and spinal cord. This part of the brain mediates the nausea and vomiting response if toxins are detected in the bloodstream. The hypothesis is that trauma can directly irritate this region of the brain and thus results in nausea. Some also believe that there is a component of concussion of the vestibular (balance) organ that can lead to the longer-lasting feeling of nausea and imbalance.

80. How long does post-concussive syndrome last?

The duration of symptoms is generally related to the severity of the initial injury, although this is not a hard-and-fast rule. Individuals who completely lose consciousness can recover fully from a neurological standpoint almost immediately, whereas some people who suffer mild trauma can have symptoms that last for weeks. The severity of the injury is usually measured not in terms of length of a loss of consciousness but rather in severity of cognitive problems (like concentration or memory difficulty), headache, or fatigue.

81. What is second-impact syndrome?

Second-impact syndrome (SIS) is a serious sequence of traumatic events to the brain that can potentially lead to serious, even fatal, injuries. Usually seen in the context of athletics, this syndrome can occur any time that trauma to the head occurs repeatedly in a short amount of time. If an individual suffers a mild head injury, then receives a second injury before the brain has had a chance to recover fully from the initial insult, then a rapid and catastrophic increase of pressure within the skull can result. The effects from this increased pressure can include paralysis, lifelong physical or mental disability, and even death.

Consultation with a health care provider following head trauma is essential in preventing SIS. At the time of publication of this text, there have been no reported cases of fatalities due to SIS when a physician was consulted following the first injury.

Consultation with a health care provider following head trauma is essential in preventing SIS.

82. When can I start playing sports or being active again?

A detailed physical and neurological exam provides the most important information in determining when it is safe to return to contact sports or other physical activity. In general, a mild concussion requires at least one week of being symptom free. The determination of what constitutes "symptom free" can be difficult to determine, and sophisticated neuropsychological testing may be needed to evaluate cognitive function precisely. The nature of the sports being played, contact versus non-contact sports, also determines the sports-free period. Mild head injuries incurred in contact sports often do not get any in-hospital assessment or imaging, and therefore may be underdiagnosed.

PART TEN

Long-Term Consequences of Head Injury

What sort of neurological problems are expected following a brain injury?

What kinds of cognitive problems can brain injury cause?

How much functioning will I regain?

More . . .

83. What sort of neurological problems are expected following a brain injury?

Certain parts of the brain are responsible for controlling specific actions. The type of physical dysfunction that might be caused by a traumatic brain injury depends on the location of the trauma within the brain.

The motor strip is located on the frontal lobe of the brain. Each half, or hemisphere, of the brain has a motor strip that controls voluntary movement on the other side of the body (i.e., the motor strip on the left frontal lobe controls movement on the right side of the body and vice versa). Damage to the motor strip may result in weakness, or even paralysis, of the other side of the body.

Many parts of the brain are required for the complete processing and integration of visual information.

The occipital lobe is located in the back of the brain and is responsible for processing visual information. Damage to the occipital lobe can result in blindness, visual illusions, or inability to read. Many parts of the brain are required for the complete processing and integration of visual information. The language areas (Broca's area and Wernicke's area) are located in the left hemisphere in most people. Damage to these areas can result in problems with understanding language, speaking, or both.

The parietal lobes are responsible for integrating the information from all the other parts of the brain. Sensory information (touch, sense of the position of limbs in space, temperature) is integrated with visual information from the occipital lobes and sounds from the temporal lobes. Damage to the parietal lobe can result in visual perception difficulty, poor hand-eye coordination, or lack of awareness of the body in space, to name a few.

Epilepsy

From the Greek word for seizure, epilepsy is the condition of persistent, if intermittent, unprovoked seizure; it may develop after a head trauma, although a single seizure in the acute period after the trauma need not mean that the patient will develop epilepsy thereafter.

84. Can a brain injury cause epilepsy?

Traumatic brain injury is a well-known cause of **epilepsy**. Seizures can develop immediately after an injury to the brain, or they can develop some time later, sometimes several months following the initial trauma. As a general rule, the risk of developing a seizure disorder is related to the severity of the injury.

A seizure is an uncontrolled electrical discharge that circulates through the brain. There are many types of seizures, but the most common type of seizure seen in the setting of traumatic brain injury is a generalized seizure (also referred to as grand mal or tonic-clonic). Seizures are dangerous because an individual who is seizing is unaware of the environment, lose control of the body, and may initiate movements that can result in serious injury (i.e., falling down, knocking furniture over onto him- or herself, choking on saliva or vomit). A seizure that lasts for more than a few minutes can result in permanent brain damage or even death.

It is not uncommon for an individual who has an injury to the brain to suffer a seizure immediately afterwards. Some individuals suffer only one seizure as a result of the trauma, while others will develop lifelong seizures as a result of their injury. As a rule of thumb, early seizures are less likely to result in a permanent seizure disorder than late ones.

85. What kinds of cognitive problems can head injury cause?

Difficulty with memory is the most common cognitive problem that people experience after a head injury. Individuals who suffer severe injuries to the brain can suffer from a condition known as "retrograde amnesia." Persons with retrograde amnesia suffer the loss of memory backward in time to a point prior to the injury, meaning that information that was previously able to be recalled is now lost following the injury. The details of the specific type of brain damage that causes this type of amnesia is not known, but it probably involves the temporal lobes and hippocampus.

Many individuals will suffer from a period of posttraumatic amnesia following an episode of unconsciousness.

Many individuals will suffer from a period of posttraumatic amnesia following an episode of unconsciousness. As recovery progresses, the survivor usually notices an increased ability to recall events prior to the injury, although in some cases the memory is permanently erased.

Community living skills, domestic duties, communication, money management, transportation, and social skills may require retraining. In the case of severe injuries, the ability to make important financial or medical decisions, to comply with medical advice, to give informed consent, or to make life decisions may be impaired. A court order to appoint a guardian or administrator for the patient may be required. The laws governing this area vary from state to state. Neuropsychological testing may help characterize the extent of any cognitive disability resulting from the injury. Information from these tests can be helpful in determining what activities are likely to be problematic and what individualized strategies can be employed to help survivors and their families compensate.

Angela's comments:

For me the hugest issue was I felt like I lost the brilliance I once had. Things used to come so easy to me, but I thought that other people who weren't as quick as I was were just lazy or not trying. I now know better. My memory is still unreliable. I have to write things down to be able to remember them. I used to love learning language, and still do, but it was very hard for me to learn languages after my injury.

86. Can brain injury cause Alzheimer's disease or Parkinson's disease?

There does appear to be an increased risk of developing Alzheimer's disease with head injury, and to a lesser extent, Parkinson's disease. The risk of developing these illnesses is increased the more severe and the more frequent the trauma to the brain is. Researchers have noticed an increased incidence of these forms of dementia in patients with head injury, but the cause is not known. The risk of developing Parkinson's disease increases eightfold for patients who require hospitalization for their brain injury, and it is elevenfold for patients who suffer a severe TBI. The great boxer Muhammad Ali now has early-onset Parkinson's disease that is believed to have been caused by the repeated head trauma he suffered during his professional boxing career. Studies of professional football players suggest that there may be a genetic predisposition to developing posttraumatic Alzheimer's disease, but this is preliminary, though intriguing, information.

87. Can brain injury cause depression?

Mood and anxiety disorders are frequent complications for patients who have had traumatic brain injury. Among patients with moderate to severe TBI, some studies have found the incidence of major depressive disorder to be as high as 50%. TBI survivors are also at increased lifetime risk of depression. The reason for this increased prevalence of serious depression in TBI survivors is currently the subject of intense research. Some signs of depression are decreased enjoyment in activities that were previously enjoyable, decreased appetite, excessive sleepiness, insomnia, or social withdrawal. Depression is a serious and potentially life-threatening condition. It is important to watch closely for the signs of a depressive episode and seek medical attention if it is suspected.

Depression is a serious and potentially life-threatening condition.

88. Will I be able to go back to work?

Although each individual's injury is different in extent and nature, TBI survivors frequently rejoin the workforce. If possible, return to work is an important goal, as it contributes to satisfaction and quality of life.

In many cases, TBI survivors have an underappreciation of their cognitive deficits and can perform poorly if pressured to return to work or school too early. Professional assessment and close monitoring are essential, particularly in the early stages of reentry into the workforce. Vocational rehabilitation is available throughout the United States for persons with mental, physical, or emotional disabilities. Services such as vocational education, counseling, job placement services, technological aides, and physical and/or mental restoration all fall under the general category of occupational rehabilitation. Be sure to check with your health care provider or social worker to determine what if any of these services might be applicable to your situation.

89. Is there a way to determine the severity of a brain injury?

Most people who suffer traumatic brain injuries fall into the mild traumatic brain injury (TBI) category. These injuries rarely require inpatient rehabilitation, but up to 10% of patients report persistent problems more than six months after an injury.

Patients with moderate and severe injuries display a very broad range of possible outcomes. It is not possible to predict what the long-term recovery will be like in the initial weeks following the trauma. Even patients with severe injuries and initially dire prognoses can successfully return to gainful employment and normal community life.

It is not possible to predict what the long-term recovery will be like in the initial weeks following the trauma.

The duration of posttraumatic amnesia (PTA) is the best indicator of the severity of cognitive and functional deficits following brain injury. The period of PTA is defined as the period of time after TBI during which the brain is unable to form continuous day-to-day memory. The longer the period of PTA, the worse the ultimate deficits are. Most patients with PTA of less than two weeks tend to have fairly good functional outcome, and those with durations longer than six weeks are more profoundly affected.

The Glasgow Coma Scale (GCS) is a standardized scale that is used to grade the level of consciousness or ability to interact with the environment. The GCS is commonly used in the setting of traumatic brain injury, but it is more useful in terms of predicting survival from an injury more than degree of functional recovery.

90. How much function will I regain?

This is perhaps the most commonly asked and most difficult question to answer. It is impossible to predict how much function will be regained following a traumatic brain injury, particularly in the weeks following the initial event. Generally speaking, the more severe the initial deficit, the more profound the ultimate dysfunction will be. What we do know is that for most people, 90% of the total recovery will be reached by the one-year anniversary of the injury. How long it takes to reach that 90% and what the specific functions will be are impossible to predict.

Also, recovery means different things to different patients and their families. Recovery is defined as any improvement, but more important to most patients and their families is the functional recovery. Functional recovery to a level of independence with feeding and caring for oneself is important. Other patients may consider recovery as improvement to a point where they are able to work. The expectations need to be matched with the degree of injury. For example, recovery from severe head injury and deep coma to a state where a patient can interact with the environment would be considered a dramatic recovery. Even if such a patient were to remain on lifelong supportive care but could interact with family and loved ones, this would be a good outcome. In this case independence should not be the expectation.

PART ELEVEN

Rehabilitation after Head Trauma and Brain Injury

How long does it take to recover from a head injury?

What kinds of problems can I expect during rehabilitation?

What can be done to help with mood and personality changes caused by brain injury?

More . . .

91. How long does it take to recover from a head injury?

The time required for recovery following trauma is highly variable, ranging from a few minutes, in the case of a minor injury, to permanent and profound disability. Generally speaking, the more severe the injury, the longer recovery will take, although it is impossible to predict how much recovery an individual will make or how long it will take. In the case of severe brain injury, recovery is measured in terms of weeks and months, not days or hours. Rehabilitation is mentally and physically exhausting for both patients and their families. Clinicians have created the Glasgow outcome scale (Table 6) to categorize uniformly how head injury patients recover.

Table 6. Glasgow Outcome Scale

Category	Definition
Good outcome	Implies resumption of normal life; may be minor neurological and/or psychological deficits
Moderately disabled (disabled but independent)	Able to work in a sheltered environment and travel by public transportation
Severely disabled (conscious but not independent)	Dependent for daily support by reason of mental or physical disability or both
Persistent vegetative state	Unresponsive and speechless for weeks or months or until death; may have sleep-wake cycles after 2-3 weeks

92. How does the brain recover lost abilities?

The precise mechanisms by which the brain repairs itself following injury are the subject of active research. Traditionally, physicians were taught that once the human brain reaches maturity, further growth or repair is not possible. We now know that this is not true, and a limited amount of regrowth and reorganization following trauma is possible, even in the adult brain. The reacquisition of lost abilities may come as a result of uninjured parts of the brain taking on new responsibilities and developing new connections to compensate for the function lost by the damaged part of the brain. The capacity to do so is very limited in adults, and most areas of the brain that are damaged lead to permanent loss of function associated with that area. Recovery occurs for two main reasons in adults. One, many brain functions are mediated by multiple brain areas, and the loss of one area doesn't necessarily mean the function will be lost. Also, the cells that make up brain tissue can be injured (ischemic from low blood flow) or killed (infracted). When recovery occurs, it can happen from medical/surgical efforts to prevent injured brain tissue from dying. It's also possible that neural stem cells may migrate to the area of damage and attempt to repopulate the traumatized territory with new brain tissue. As researchers begin to unlock the secrets of how this growth or reorganization occurs, they may be able to facilitate this process and develop more effective therapies for traumatic brain injuries.

> *A limited amount of regrowth and reorganization following trauma is possible, even in the adult brain.*

Angela's comments:

While the major symptoms of my TBI area are definitely milder than they initially were, I still have problems with learning and memory. I also occasionally get migraine pains in my temples, but reading this answer, I am hopeful that my brain will continue to reorganize itself to compensate for areas lost in my injury.

93. What are the objectives of rehabilitation?

The primary goals of rehabilitation from a brain injury are to restore lost function. Many people think of rehabilitation in terms of physical ability, but rehabilitation should also help people to function more independently. During rehabilitation, a patient may learn physical exercises or how to use specialized tools to augment physical movements, and family members may learn how to help the patient and modify the living environment to facilitate independent life. Many different types of rehabilitation may be employed to achieve the goal of maximizing function.

Therapists can use tools or techniques to help people who cannot speak find alternative ways to communicate.

Speech therapy refers broadly to learning techniques that are used to facilitate communication. Speech therapy may include exercises to retrain or strengthen muscles involved in speech, breathing, chewing, or swallowing. A speech therapist can also train the brain to understand words and gestures and learn new ways to concentrate and process information. Therapists can use tools or techniques to help people who cannot speak find alternative ways to communicate.

94. What kinds of problems can I expect during rehabilitation?

The most important thing to remember when going through rehabilitation from a neurological injury is that progress is measured on the scale of weeks and months and not hours or days. Rehabilitation is a long and arduous process that requires hard work, perseverance, and above all patience on the part of the patient and the entire support network.

The specific problems that arise are difficult to predict because they depend on the severity and spectrum of disabilities that exist following the injury. In general, the more profound the dysfunction the more potential there is for unexpected problems to arise. Talk to your health care provider to find out what specific problems to expect and how you can identify them before they get out of hand.

95. How does a severely brain-injured individual receive nourishment?

Injuries to the central nervous system can impair the nerves that control the chewing (lips, cheeks, tongue, jaw) and the safe swallowing of food and liquid. In the initial stages of recovery, the patient is likely to receive water and essential electrolytes intravenously. If the individual is unable to safely receive food or water after more than a few days, then a feeding tube can be placed into the stomach, either temporarily through the esophagus (via the nose or mouth) or surgically through the abdominal wall. A surgical feeding tube can remain in place for many months or years and is an effective way to deliver food and hydration to a disabled brain injury survivor. These feeding tubes can be permanent or temporary if the individual recovers the ability to swallow safely over time.

96. Can a person's balance be affected by traumatic brain injury?

Trouble with balance and equilibrium is very common following traumatic brain injury. Many parts of the brain need to function and be integrated for the equilibrium sense to operate. The inner ear is where the balance center, called the vestibular apparatus, is located. The visual system is also crucial to the sense of balance and equilibrium. Any derangement in the vestibular apparatus, the visual apparatus, or their interconnections can result in balance problems.

Of course, the muscles that control the voluntary movements of the body might be weakened due to damage to the motor cortex, the part of the brain that controls the muscles of the body. If that is the case, a person may have a normally functioning sense of balance but be unable to initiate the movements quickly or forcefully enough to correct posture or balance. The functional outcome of a disorder like this is a fall or balance difficulty, even though a different part of the brain is affected from the visual or vestibular apparatuses.

97. What is midline shift syndrome?

Midline shift syndrome is a posttraumatic vision syndrome that affects the brain's ability to process balance and spatial orientation information. Patients experience a constant sense of disequilibrium, an inappropriate posture, unequal weight distribution on their feet, dysfunctional gait, and a directional drift. Patients frequently say that the world seems tilted, that walls are slanted, or that the walls and ceiling are closing in on them.

Consultation with a balance expert, such as an otolaryngologist or a neurolotologist, is essential because although there are effective therapies for this condition (such as yoked prism reorientation), other causes for disequilibrium must be ruled out.

98. What can be done to help with mood and personality changes caused by brain injury?

Dramatic mood swings, also called emotional lability, and behavioral disturbances, are common following severe brain injury. Medical therapies are available, usually under the care of a specialist (such as a neuropsychiatrist), to stabilize the disposition of TBI survivors who display behavioral problems. Other, nonmedical interventions are used as well. Cognitive-behavioral therapy allows an individual to increase awareness of when a mood change might be occurring, and for that person to initiate alternate behaviors that might mitigate the severity or impact of the abnormal behavior.

Behavioral changes have the very serious potential impact of alienating family and friends. Ignorance and misconceptions about the effects of TBI by family members, coworkers, and even health care professionals can exacerbate the problem. It is important for family members to be aware of the potential for behavioral disturbances and act quickly to seek help for their loved one.

99. What is the relationship between brain injury and drug or alcohol addiction?

It is estimated that up to 50% of civilian traumatic brain injuries in adults are intoxicated at the time of injury. Head injuries are two to four times more common in alcoholics than in the general population. Alcoholics who have sustained head injuries perform significantly more poorly on psychometric tests than uninjured alcoholics. Drug and alcohol abuse places users at increased risk for brain injury, and these individuals appear to suffer more deleterious effects than nonusers with similar injuries.

In addition, severe brain injury can disrupt the normal functioning of the frontal lobes of the brain. The frontal lobes are responsible for exercising judgment and restraint. Survivors of TBI often display impulsiveness and impaired judgment. When coupled with the increased incidence of psychiatric problems (such as anxiety, posttraumatic stress disorder, and depression), these individuals are at increased risk of developing alcohol or drug addiction.

Drug and alcohol abuse places users at increased risk for brain injury.

100. Can severe head injury cause changes in personality?

Personality changes can occur, and they can be pronounced, particularly when the injury is severe. Several clinically recognized syndromes describe changes in personality following brain trauma. Orbitofrontal syndrome is characterized by disinhibition, poor judgment, inappropriate behavior, and impulsivity. Individuals with dorsolateral prefrontal syndrome display apathy, psychomotor slowing, and lack of motivation. The extent and nature of personality change, if any, is impossible to predict. Through more sophisticated neuropsychological testing, scientists are discovering that even moderately severe head injuries can result in very subtle changes in cognitive and psychological behavior. Our understanding of the spectrum of derangements that can occur following brain trauma is evolving. Severe and permanent personality changes do occur following brain injury, and generally speaking, the more severe the injury, the more profound the change in personality may be.

Appendix

Brain Injury Association of America
1608 Spring Hill Road
Suite 110
Vienna, VA 22182
(703) 761-0750
www.biausa.org
Founded in 1980, BIAA is a national organization that provides support and education for those affected by a brain injury. For information and resources, call their Information Center at (800) 444-6443.

National Center for Injury Prevention and Control
Mailstop F41
4770 Buford Highway NE
Atlanta, GA 30341-3724
(800) CDC-INFO (1-800-232-4636)
cdcinfo@cdc.gov
www.cdc.gov/ncipc/tbi/TBI.htm
An organization in the Centers for Disease Control and Prevention, part of the Department of Health and Human Services, the Center's mission is to promote healthy living for all people. This Web site is a valuable source for clearly written facts on traumatic brain injury.

Brain Injury Society
1901 Avenue N
Suite 5E
Brooklyn, NY 11230
(718) 645-4401
www.bisociety.org
The Brain Injury Society is dedicated to providing techniques to those suffering from a brain injury. Focusing on a speedy response, the organization works to maximize the potential for recovery. They feature support groups, links to press releases and current news, and more information on brain injuries.

TraumaticBrainInjury.com
Two Penn Center Plaza
Suite 1705
Philadelphia, PA 19102-1865
www.traumaticbraininjury.com
This educational site has in-depth information pertaining to symptoms, treatment, and understanding brain injuries. It also provides legal resources and a video library.

Glossary

B

Brain stem: The part of the central nervous system responsible for a number of "unconscious" activities, including breathing, heart rate, wakefulness, and sleep.

C

Central nervous system (CNS): Pertaining to the brain and spinal cord.

Cerebellum: Part of the brain located at the back of the head, under the cerebrum and in front of the brain stem. Controls balance and coordination, affecting movements of the same side of the body.

Cerebral aneurysm: From the Greek for "widening," an aneurysm is a pathological widening of a blood vessel that can be either local, like a blister or "berry" aneurysm, or gradual, called "fusiform." Aneurysms can be congenital or result from connective tissue disorders, infection in the cerebral vessels, or hypertension; these widenings of vessels are at increased risk of spontaneous hemorrhage, a potentially fatal event.

Cerebral edema: Brain swelling that may result from increased vascular permeability or increased intraparenchymal particle content due to the failure of normal brain metabolism and the build-up of metabolic by-products.

Cerebrospinal fluid (CSF): Produced by a portion of the brain called the choroid plexus as a filtrate of the blood, cerebrospinal fluid (also commonly called "spinal fluid") both mechanically buffers the brain from trauma and clears its metabolites; imbalance of its production, transmission, or reabsorption is called "hydrocephalus."

Computed tomography (CT) scan: A scan produced by computer analysis of a long series of x-rays, a CT scan evaluates the relative densities of objects. In CT scans of the brain, the objects are usually compared to the normal brain; for example, acute blood clots are more dense ("hyperdense") in comparison to normal brain tissue. This is the most common screening radiographic study in the context of acute injury.

Consciousness: Emerging from a combination of a part of the brain stem that causes overall arousal and the function of both cerebral hemispheres, consciousness is the state of both awareness of the world and active volition in carrying out actions; it is most easily manifested clinically by the capacity to understand verbal or written cues and obey them.

Cortex: The outer surface of the cerebral hemispheres; often called the gray matter.

Cranial nerves: Nerves that arise from the base of the brain or the brain stem that provide sensory and motor functions to the eyes, nose, ears, tongue, and face.

Craniectomy: A surgical "cutting" of an opening into the skull, after which the bone is not returned to the patient's skull.

D

Deep vein thrombosis (DVT): Clotting that can occur within the deep veins of the body, especially when someone is immobilized or more prone to coagulation by systemic inflammation.

Dura mater: The outermost covering of the brain, a tough and fibrous membrane found immediately under the skull; injuries are often compared to this membrane for location: for example, epidural (on or outside the dura) and subdural (beneath the dura).

E

Electroencephalogram (EEG): Like an electrocardiogram that measures the electrical signals of the heart, an EEG measures the electrical activity of the brain; it can be used to detect the presence of absence (for example, in brain death) of normal electrical activity or to detect the abnormal activity of seizure.

Epilepsy: From the Greek word for seizure, epilepsy is the condition of persistent, if intermittent, unprovoked seizure; it may develop after a head trauma, although a single seizure in the acute period after the trauma need not mean that the patient will develop epilepsy thereafter.

Euthanasia: From a Greek term meaning "dying well," euthanasia is currently used to describe a set of practices that occupy a difficult medico-legal position and, ideally, produce a gentle and easy death in those who are deathly ill or debilitated without hope of recovery.

F

Falx cerebri: From the Latin for "scythe of the brain," the falx is a fold of dura mater that divides the left and right cerebral hemispheres from one another.

Fontanelles: Commonly called "soft spots," the fontanelles are the portions of the skull not yet ossified in infants; they usually fuse between the first and second years of life.

Foramen magnum: From Latin, meaning "the great hole," the foramen magnum is the hole at the base of the skull through which the spinal cord emerges.

Fourth ventricle: One of the spinal fluid pathways in the midline of the brain, between the brain stem and the cerebellum.

Frontal lobe: The anterior (toward the face) area in the cerebral hemisphere involved in emotion, thought, reasoning, and behavior.

G

Glasgow Coma Scale (GCS): A scale for the evaluation of consciousness, it is a fifteen-point scale that involves three separate areas: eye opening, verbal response, and motor activity; a functional person in the normal state of health has a score of fifteen; difficulty with eye opening, verbal expression, and motor responses results in lower scores. At or below a score of eight, the patient may require the assistance of a ventilator.

H

Head trauma: An injury to the head, which would include the brain, but could also be used to describe injury to the face and skull.

Hematoma: A technical term for a blood clot; hematomas are often localized to the spaces either immediately inside the outer covering of the brain ("epidural hematoma") or beneath it ("subdural hematoma").

Hemisphere: One of the two halves of the cerebrum or cerebellum.

Herniation: The forced passage of one anatomical structure across a normal anatomical barrier, as in an abdominal hernia; herniation in the central nervous system can result in injury both to the structure forced across the barrier and the structure occupying the space into which it is forced; the most notorious example is uncal herniation, in which the middle part of the temporal lobe herniates through the opening of the tentorium cerebelli and crushes the brain stem, resulting in severe injury.

Hydrocephalus: The imbalance of the production, transmission, or reabsorption of cerebrospinal fluid; may occur in the context of acute injury due to the blockage of fluid flow from its point of production inside the brain to its point of absorption around the outside of the brain and spine; may require temporary drainage with an external drain or permanent, indwelling drainage with a ventriculoperitoneal shunt.

I

Intracranial pressure (ICP): The pressure within the fixed cranial vault that is produced by the relative volumes of brain, blood, cerebrospinal fluid, and "other" materials, such as tumor or infection; it can be measured with transcranial devices such as a pressure transducer or even a drain that can also reduce the intracranial volume of the cerebrospinal fluid and, indirectly, the total intracranial pressure.

L

Lateral ventricles: The two elongated, curved openings in each cerebral hemisphere connecting with two slit-like openings in the center of the brain.

M

Magnetic resonance imaging (MRI) scan: A scan produced by comparison of magnetic properties; various methods of analysis are used, resulting in different imaging appearances for objects that are magnetic or not; can demonstrate injuries to the brain not visible on CT scan.

Monro-Kellie Doctrine: The principle of skull contents being fixed, meaning that the addition of a space-occupying legion will lead to compression of the brain because an adult skull cannot expand.

N

Neurological deficit: Partial or complete loss of muscle strength, sensation, or other brain functions; may be temporary or permanent.

Neurological examination: Part of the physical examination testing general intellectual function, speech, motor function, memory, sensation, reflexes, and cranial nerve functions.

Neurosurgeon: A surgical specialist whose area of concentration includes the management and treatment of acute intracranial and spinal injuries.

O

Occipital lobe: The area in the cerebral hemispheres that interprets visual images as well as the meaning of written words.

P

Parietal lobe: The area in the cerebral hemispheres that controls sensory and motor information.

Physical therapy: Therapy aimed at recovery from weakness, loss of coordination, or limited endurance.

Positron emission tomography (PET) scan: A nuclear medicine study that uses the detection of radio-labeled metabolic by-products; it is often used to detect normal or abnormal metabolism as is found in the context of injury and neoplasm.

Prognosis: The long-term outlook for survival and recovery based upon the patient's current status and the anticipated effect of available treatments.

S

Subcortical: A term used to describe the part of the brain that is not on the surface.

T

Temporal lobe: The area in the cerebral hemispheres that contains both the auditory and visual pathways and the interpretation of sounds and spoken language for long-term memory.

Tentorium cerebelli: From the Latin for "the tent of the cerebellum," the tentorium is a fold of the dura that covers the cerebellum and divides it from the cerebrum; it has a hole in the middle of it through which the brain stem passes called the "incisura tentorii."

Third ventricle: A spinal fluid-filled space in the center of the brain in communication with the lateral ventricles.

V

Ventilator: A machine designed to support a patient's airway and provide needed oxygen; oxygen can be passed temporarily through a tube down the patient's throat, called an endotracheal tube, or through a permanent, surgical airway called a tracheostomy.

Ventricle: From Latin for "little belly," a ventricle is a fluid-filled space. The brain has four separate spaces within it called ventricles, all of which are filled with cerebrospinal fluid. Two of these spaces are referred to as "lateral ventricles," with one in each hemisphere of the brain. One is called the "third ventricle," which is in the very middle of the brain and into which the lateral ventricles drain their cerebrospinal fluid. Finally, there is also the so-called fourth ventricle, which is also in the midline but at the base of the brain and into which the third ventricle itself drains and from which the spinal fluid drains to the space around the spinal cord.

Index

A

abulia (como vigil), 49

acute subdural hematoma, 40

adult brain function, 11. *See also* brain function

alcohol addiction, 100–101

altered mental status, 47–49. *See also* concussion

Alzheimer's disease, 90–91

amnesia, 89, 92

anatomy, skull, 3–4

    children vs. adults, 30

aneurysms, cerebral, 43

antibiotics after brain surgery, 60–61

anti-seizure medications, 62–63

anxiety disorders, 91

arachnoid, 5

arachnoid granulations, 9

area postrema, 84–85

arteries of brain, injury to, 43–44

    middle meningeal artery, 37

    rupture (cerebral aneurysm), 43

assessing patients in hospital, 66

awake, forced after injury, 71

axons, 6

B

balance problems, 85, 99–100

bleeding risk after surgery, 60–61

blood clots. *See* hemorrhage and hematoma

blood tests, 24

blood-brain barrier, 18

blood-thinning medications, 69

bolt (for monitoring intracranial pressure), 55–56

bones of skull, 3–4. *See also* skull fracture

brain, 7–8

    artery injury, 37, 43–44

    formation of, 2

    function of, 8

    regions of, 6–8

    surface anatomy, 4–6

brain damage. *See* brain function, damage to

brain death, 49–52

    body movement during, 78

    coma vs., 50

brain function

    altered mental status, 47–49. *See also* concussion

    Alzheimer's and Parkinson's diseases, 91

    cell disruption, 15

    children vs. adults, 11

    coma. *See* coma

    complete lack of. *See* brain death

    consciousness and, 8–9. *See also* consciousness

    damage to, 88, 89

    depression, 91

    restoring. *See* recovery from injury

    symptoms of injury, 21–23

    vegetative state, 73–79

    ventricles, 9–11

brain hemorrhage. *See* hemorrhage and hematoma

brain herniation, 19–20. *See also* brain swelling

    defined, 17

    types of, 19–20

brain injury, 14–15

    diagnosing, 70–71

    fever from, 70

    herniation. *See* brain herniation

    hospitalization, 65–71

    long-term consequences, 87–93

    measuring severity of, 91. *See also* Glasgow Coma Scale (GCS)

    Monro-Kellie doctrine, 17

prevention against. *See* prevention against injury

recovery from. *See* recovery from injury

rehabilitation, 95–101

signs and symptoms of, 21–23

skull protection and contribution, 16–17

swelling. *See* brain swelling

trauma without, 14. *See also* head trauma

traumatic (TBI), 82, 88–89, 91–92

ventilator support, 54–55

Brain Injury Association of America, 103

Brain Injury Society, 103

brain scans. *See* CT scans; MRI scans

brain stem
defined, 5
effects of injury to, 23
function of, 6

brain surgeon (neurosurgeon)
defined, 8
in intensive care unit, 67
when necessary, 27

brain swelling, 17–19
hospitalization for, 68
monitoring, 55–57
treatment for, 18, 57–59, 61–62

Broca's area, 88

bruising. *See* hemorrhage and hematoma

buffering against brain swelling, 19

C

carbon dioxide in blood, 54

cardiac activity after brain death, 51–52

care, withdrawing, 78–79

carotid artery. *See* arteries of brain, injury to

catheter (drainage tube). *See also* surgery
after surgery, 62
for hydrocephalus, 10, 42
infection from, 11
risks of, 60
ventricular drain, 56–57

causes of head trauma in kids, 30

cell disruption, 15

central herniation, 19–20

central nervous system (CNS), formation of, 2

cerebellum, 4
defined, 2
effects of injury to, 23
function of, 6

cerebral aneurysms, 43

cerebral edema, defined, 17

cerebrospinal fluid, 9–10. *See also* surgery
buildup of (hydrocephalus)
catheter for, 10, 42
defined, 10
leakage of, 11, 36
ventricular drain, 56–57

children vs. adults, 26
brain function in, 11
skull anatomy, 30

chronic subdural hematoma, 40

clots (blood). *See* hemorrhage and hematoma

CNS (central nervous system), formation of, 2

coagulation abnormalities, 24, 61

cognitive problems following head injury, 89–90

cognitive-behavioral therapy, 100

coma, 45–52, 74. *See also* consciousness (being awake); vegetative state
abulia (como vigil), 49
altered mental status vs. unconsciousness, 47–49
brain death, 49–52
diffuse axonal injury (DAI), 49–50
evaluating comatose patients. *See also* consciousness (being awake)
Glasgow Coma Scale (GCS), 46–47, 74, 93
inducing, 8, 58
movement of body during, 75–76
treatment for, 77

comatose patients, evaluating, 23

como vigil (abulia), 49

compression of brain. *See* brain swelling

computed tomography. *See* CT scans

concussion, 81–86
   defined, 81
   sleeping after, 71

consciousness (being awake). *See also*
   coma
   brain regions responsible for, 8–9
   concussion and, 82
   defined, 8
   forced, after injury, 71
   keeping patient unconscious, 8–9, 58
   vegetative state, 73–79

consultation with neurosurgeon
   defined, 8
   in intensive care unit, 67
   when necessary, 27

contusions, intracerebral, 41

cortex, 5, 6

counter-coup injury, 16

coup injury, 16

cranial nerves, defined, 3

craniectomy, 59, 60–62

cranioplasty, 59

cribriform plate fracture, 36

CT scans, 24–26, 70
   detecting intracerebral hematomas,
     41
   diagnosing coma or vegetative state,
     77
   diffuse axonal injury (DAI), 50

cytotoxic processes, defined, 18

D

DAI (diffuse axonal injury), 49–50

death after withdrawal of care, 79

decompressive craniectomy, 61–62

deep vein thrombosis (DVT), 69–70

dementia, 90–91

depressed skull fractures, 34

depression, brain injury and, 91

diagnosing
   brain death, 50–51
   coma or vegetative state, 77–78
   head injury, tests for, 24–27

post-concussive syndrome, 83
   trauma and injury, 21–23, 70–71

diffuse axonal injury (DAI), 49–50

disabled (Glasgow outcome scale), 96

dissections, lumen, 44

donation of bodily organs, 52

drainage tube (catheter). *See* catheter
   (drainage tube)

draining cerebrospinal fluid, 10

drug addiction, 100–101

drugs (illicit), checking for, 24

drugs (legal). *See* medications

dura mater, defined, 5

DVT (deep vein thrombosis), 69–70

dysfunction. *See* brain function

E

electroencephalograms (EEG), defined,
   77–78

emotional liability, 100

employment following head injury,
   91–92

epidural hematoma, 37–39
   operative treatment for, 59–60

epidural space, 5, 37

epilepsy, caused by brain injury, 88–89

epinephrine, 84

euthanasia, withdrawing care vs., 79

evaluation of head injury, 23–27

eye category, Glasgow Coma Scale, 46

F

falls, as cause of injury, 30

falx cerebri, defined, 3

feeding severely brain–injured
   individuals, 98–99

fetal development of brain and skull, 2

fever, from brain injury, 70

fluid compartments in brain. *See*
   ventricles

fluid of spine. *See* cerebrospinal fluid

fontanelles, 30
   defined, 2
   intraventricular hemorrhage, 42

foramen magnum, defined, 3

formation of brain and skull, 2
fourth ventricle, defined, 9. *See also*
  ventricles
fractures (skull), 34–36
  expansion of, in children, 31
  operations for, 35
frontal bone, 3
frontal lobe, 5
  effects of injury to, 22
  function of, 6
  judgment impairment after injury,
    100–101
frontal sinus, fracture of, 35, 59
function, brain
  altered mental status, 47–49. *See also*
    concussion
  Alzheimer's and Parkinson's diseases,
    91
  cell disruption, 15
  children vs. adults, 11
  coma. *See* coma
  complete lack of. *See* brain death
  consciousness and, 8–9. *See also*
    consciousness
  damage to, 88, 89
  depression, 91
  restoring. *See* recovery from injury
  symptoms of injury, 21–23
  vegetative state, 73–79
  ventricles, 9–11
function, skull, 3
functional recovery, defined, 93

G

Glasgow Coma Scale (GCS), 46–47,
  74, 93
Glasgow outcome scale, 96
gray matter. *See* cortex
gyri, 4

H

head injury, 23. *See also* brain injury
  diffuse axonal injury (DAI), 49–50
  hospitalization after, 65–71
  long-term consequences, 87–93

physical exam for, 21
rehabilitation, 95–101
ventilator support, 54–55
head trauma, 13–27
  arterial injury, 37, 43–44
  causes of, 15
  in children, common causes of, 30
  children vs. adults, 26
  concussion, 81–86
  defined, 13
  epidural hematoma, 37–39
  evaluation (in hospital), 23–27
  hemorrhage and, 37
  intracerebral hematomas
    (intracerebral contusions), 41
  intraventricular hemorrhage, 42
  Monro-Kellie doctrine, 17
  recovery from. *See* recovery from
    injury
  rehabilitation, 95–101
  scalp laceration, 34
  signs and symptoms of, 21–23
  skull fracture, 31, 34–36
  subarachnoid hemorrhage (SAH), 43
  subdural hematoma (SDH), 39–41
  treatment. *See* treatment
  when to consult a neurosurgeon, 27
head/brain injury. *See* brain injury
hearing during vegetative state, 76
hearing loss, 36
heart activity after brain death, 51–52
helmets, wearing, 30
hematoma, defined, 26. *See also*
    hemorrhage and hematoma
hemispheres, 4
  skull anatomy and, 3
hemorrhage and hematoma, 31, 37–43
  deep vein thrombosis (DVT), 69–70
  defined, 26
  epidural hematoma, 37–39
  intracerebral hematomas
    (intracerebral contusions), 41
  intraventricular hemorrhage, 42
  operative treatment for, 59–60
  subarachnoid hemorrhage (SAH), 43
  subdural hematoma (SDH), 39–41

herniation. *See* brain herniation
hospitalization, 65–71
  deep vein thrombosis (DVT), 69–70
  goals of, 68
  intensive care unit, 66–67
  pain treatment, 68–69
  patient monitoring and assessment, 66
hydrocephalus
  catheter for, 10, 42
  defined, 10
hyperventilation, 18

I

ICP (intracranial pressure), 55–57. *See also* brain swelling
ICU (intensive care unit), 66–67
immobilized patients, 69
impulsiveness after injury, 100–101
inducing coma, 8, 58
infection
  of brain fluid, 10
  from brain surgery, risk of, 60–61
  from catheter, 11
initial operation period, after injury, 67
injury. *See also* head trauma
  to arteries, 37, 43–44
  brain herniation. *See* brain herniation
  brain swelling. *See* brain herniation
  diffuse axonal injury (DAI), 49–50
  evaluation (in hospital), 23–27
  fever from brain injury, 70
  hospitalization after, 65–71
  long-term consequences, 87–93
  measuring severity of, 91. *See also* Glasgow Coma Scale (GCS)
  Monro-Kellie doctrine, 17
  prevention against. *See* prevention against injury
  recovery from. *See* recovery from injury
  rehabilitation, 95–101
  signs and symptoms of, 21–23
  skull protection and contribution, 16–17

traumatic brain injury (TBI), 82
  ventilator support, 54–55
inner ear. *See* balance problems
intensive care unit, 66–67
intracerebral hematoma and contusion, 41
intracranial pressure (ICP), 55–57. *See also* brain swelling
intraventricular hemorrhage, 42

J

judgment impairment after injury, 100–101

L

laceration, scalp, 34
language processing, 88
lateral ventricles, defined, 9. *See also* ventricles
leakage of cerebrospinal fluid, 11, 36
loss of consciousness, 47–49. *See also* consciousness (being awake)
lucid interval, 38
lumen, tears of, 44

M

magnetic resonance imaging. *See* MRI scans
malignant edema, 18
medications
  antibiotics after brain surgery, 60–61
  blood thinners, 69
  for brain swelling, 18, 57–58
  checking blood for, 24
  in diagnosing brain death, 50–51
  pain treatment, 68–69
  sedative medications, 8–9, 58
  seizure medications, 62–63
  withdrawing care, 78–79
memory loss, 89, 92
mental status, altered, 47–49. *See also* concussion
middle meningeal artery, 37
midline shift syndrome, 99–100

mild head/brain injury, 91
  GCS score for, 47
  hospital stay for, 67
  ventilator support, 54
minimally interactive state, 75
moderate head/brain injury, 91
  GCS score for, 47
  ventilator support, 54
moderately disabled (Glasgow outcome
  scale), 96
monitoring brain swelling, 55–57
monitoring patients in hospital, 66
Monro-Kellie doctrine, 17
mood disorders, 91, 100
motor category, Glasgow Coma Scale, 46
motor strip, damage to, 88
movement after brain death, 78
movement while in coma, 75–76
MRI scans, 25–27, 70
  diagnosing coma or vegetative state, 77
  diffuse axonal injury (DAI), 50

N

National Center for Injury Prevention
  and Control, 103
nausea after concussion, 84–85
neurological deficits, defined, 8
neurological examination, defined, 55
neurological problems following injury,
  88
neurosurgeon
  defined, 8
  in intensive care unit, 67
  when necessary, 27
nourishment to severely brain–injured
  individuals, 98–99

O

occipital bone, 3
occipital lobe
  damage to, 88
  defined, 3
  effects of injury to, 23
  function of, 6
organ donation, 52
oxygen delivery to lungs, 54

P

pain treatment, 68–69
  withdrawing care and, 79
parietal lobe, 5
  damage to, 88
  effects of injury to, 22
  function of, 6
Parkinson's disease, 90–91
patient monitoring in hospital, 66
PCS. See post-concussive syndrome
PE (pulmonary embolus), 69
penetrating trauma, 15. See also head
  trauma
  protection from skull, 16
persistent vegetative state (PVS), 73–79,
  96. See also brain death; coma
  ability to hear during, 76
  treatment for, 77
  waking up from, 76
personality changes, 100, 101
PET scans, defined, 77–78
pharmaceuticals. See medications
physical exam
  for brain death, 51
  for brain swelling, 55
  for head/brain injury, 21
physical therapy, 77
pia, 5
positron emission tomography (PET)
  scans, defined, 77–78
post-concussive syndrome, 81–86
  second-impact syndrome (SIS), 85
posttraumatic amnesia (PTA), 92
posttraumatic seizure disorder, 62
prevention against injury
  buffering against brain swelling, 19
  during coma or vegetative state, 77
  fever prevention, 70
  skull as protective barrier, 19
  wearing helmets, 30
prognosis, defined, 31
protection of brain by skull, 16
PTA (posttraumatic amnesia), 92
pulmonary embolus (PE), 69
PVS. See persistent vegetative state
  (PVS)

R

recovery from injury, 93
    children vs. adults, 11, 31
    process of, 96–97
    rehabilitation, 95–101
regions of brains, 6–8
rehabilitation, 95–101
    how brain recovers, 96–97
    objectives of, 97–98
    problems during, 98
resources for further research, 103–104
respiratory support, withdrawing, 79
restoring function. *See* recovery from
    injury
reticular activating system, 8
retrograde amnesia, 89, 92
returning to work after injury, 91–92
risks of brain surgery, 60–61
ruptured brain artery, 43

S

SAH (subarachnoid hemorrhage), 43
scalp laceration, 34
scans. *See* CT scans; MRI scans
SDH (subdural hematoma), 39–41
    operative treatment for, 59–60
second-impact syndrome (SIS), 85
sedative medications, 8–9
    for brain swelling, 58
seizures, 21
    caused by brain injury, 88–89
    defined, 89
    medication for, 62–63
    posttraumatic seizure disorder, 62
sensory information processing, 88
severe head/brain injury, 91
    GCS score for, 47
    ventilator support, 54
severely disabled (Glasgow outcome
    scale), 96
severity of brain injury, 92–93
signs of trauma and injury, 21–23
SIS (second-impact syndrome), 85
skull
    anatomy of, 3–4, 30
    children vs. adults, 30

contribution to brain injury, 16–17
    formation of, 2
    function of, 3
    Monro-Kellie doctrine, 17
    operative treatment for, 59
    protection from injury, 16
    removal of sections (craniectomy), 59,
        60–62
skull fracture, 34–36
    expansion of, in children, 31
    operations for, 35
sleeping after brain injury, 71
soft spots (fontanelles), 30
    defined, 2
    intraventricular hemorrhage, 42
speech therapy, 98
spinal fluid. *See* cerebrospinal fluid
studies for head injury, 24–26
subarachnoid hemorrhage (SAH), 43
subcortical region, 7
subdural hematoma (SDH), 39–41
    operative treatment for, 59–60
subdural space, 5
subfalcine herniation, 19–20
sulci, 4
surgery
    for arterial injury, 44
    for brain swelling, 18, 59, 61–62
    for epidural hematoma, 38
    for intracerebral hematoma, 41
    risks of, 61–62
    for skull fracture, 36
    for subdural hematomas, 40
    when necessary, 59–60
swelling. *See* brain swelling
symptoms of trauma and injury, 21–23
    concussion, 82
    long-term consequences, 87–93
    post-concussive syndrome, 84–85

T

TBI (traumatic brain injury), 82
    balance problems after, 85, 99–100
    as cause of epilepsy, 88–89
    measuring severity of, 91
    returning to work after, 91–92

temporal bone, 3
    fractures of, 34, 36, 37
temporal lobe, 5
    effects of injury to, 22
    function of, 6
tentorium cerebri, defined, 3
tests for coma or vegetative state, 77–78
tests for head injury, 24–27
    CT scans. *See* CT scans
    MRI scans. *See* MRI scans
third ventricle, defined, 9. *See also*
    ventricles
tonsilar herniation, 19–20
transtentorial (uncal) herniation, 19–20
trauma. *See* head trauma; recovery from
    injury
trauma centers, 67
traumatic aneurysms, 43
traumatic brain injury (TBI), 82
    balance problems after, 85, 99–100
    as cause of epilepsy, 88–89
    measuring severity of, 91
    returning to work after, 91–92
TraumaticBrainInjury.com site, 104
treatment, 53–63. *See also* recovery from
    injury
    arterial injury, 44
    for brain swelling, 18, 55–58, 68
    coma and persistent vegetative states,
        77
    drainage after surgery, 62
    drugs. *See* medications
    for hematomas, 38, 40, 41
    hospitalization, 65–71
    minimally interactive state, 75
    for pain, 68–69
    rehabilitation, 95–101
    seizure medications, 62–63
    skull fracture surgery. *See* surgery
    surgical. *See* surgery
    withdrawing care, 78–79

U

uncal (transtentorial) herniation, 19–20
unconsciousness. *See* consciousness
    (being awake)

unresponsive patients, examining, 23.
    See also coma; consciousness (being
    awake)

V

vascular injuries, 44
vasogenic edema, defined, 18
vegetative state, 73–79, 96. *See also* brain
    death; coma
    ability to hear during, 76
    treatment for, 77
    waking up from, 76
ventilator support, 66
    after brain death, 52
    defined, 18
    when necessary, 54–55
ventricles
    children vs. adults, 30
    collapse of, to prevent swelling, 19
    defined, 2
    function of, 9–11
    intraventricular hemorrhage, 42
ventricular drain, 56–57
verbal category, Glasgow Coma Scale, 46
vertebral artery. *See* arteries of brain,
        injury to
vestibular (balance) organ, 85, 99–100
vision problems, 99–100
visual information processing, 88
vocational rehabilitation, 91

W

waking up from vegetative state, 76
weakened artery (traumatic aneurysm),
        43
Wernicke's area, 88
withdrawing care, 78–79
working after brain injury, 91–92